HOW I CURED MY
SILENT REFLUX

How I Cured My Silent Reflux

The Counterintuitive Path to Healing Acid Reflux, GERD, and Silent Reflux (LPR)

DON DANIELS

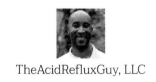

TheAcidRefluxGuy, LLC

Contents

Dedication

First and foremost, I thank God for his consistent presence and guidance throughout my life. Despite the many challenges I have outlined in this book, I have felt a consistent stewardship in my life from my marriage, to my finances, my work, and, believe it or not, my health! The sequence of events that led to my discovery of the methods, which led to my healing, and the authorship of this book could only have come from God. The approaches in this text will not heal everyone, but it's my authentic hope that they will heal you. If my fifteen years of suffering this disease leads to healing for others, then it may very well have been worth it!

I also want to say thanks to my amazing wife of fifteen years. She is tirelessly encouraging and supportive and has been a rock that I could lean on when I was struggling most. She tolerated the experimentation that ultimately led to the methods outlined in this text. Invariably, she offered unique angles that I hadn't considered. You have heard it said that a good wife is worth her weight in gold. Mine is worth twice that! For those of you that find relief using these methods, I want you to know this would not have been possible without the consistent support of my loving wife, Jenn.

Epigraph

"Once you have an understanding of the root causes of acid reflux, it is quite clear how it can be eliminated." - Don Daniels A.K.A The Acid Reflux Guy

Prologue

It felt as though I was past my breaking point. At work, my mind was constantly at war battling the pressures of leadership, constant anxiety, self-doubt, and fears of social ostracism. Over 15 years, my reflux symptoms grew to consume my every waking thought. At times, it felt as though all that was holding me together was my faith and my family.

My symptoms ultimately reached a level that was no longer manageable by medications. My nose, throat, and mouth were continuously under siege by a seemingly endless stream of mucus. The roof of my mouth, cheeks, and lips were constantly on fire. At times, I felt as though my breath could serve as a warning shot, alerting anyone who dared approach. Sadly, I was afraid to ask, for fear of confirmation and what that would do to my already fragile psyche.

I woke up each morning to headaches and spent the days finding my way through a dense cloud of brain fog. Oftentimes, I struggled to follow the thread of conversations, presentations, movie plots, etc. I struggled to stay awake when driving on long road trips often needing to start early in the day to ensure safe passage for my young family.

I grew increasingly apathetic to anything beyond my narrowing line of sight. Somewhere along the way, I lost my identity as the guy who always had something funny and witty to say. Lost was the guy whose confidence at work was based on a track record of achieving the impossible. My memory was never incredible, but when did I start comparing myself to a goldfish? Not sure... it was harder and harder to remember things.

My growing social anxiety, increasing difficulty following conversations, and articulating my thoughts were a constant challenge. I struggled with spontaneous anxiety attacks, where I broke into full body sweats as if I were playing a rigorous game of basketball in 100 degree weather! The very thought of breaking into another one of these embarrassing attacks at work, or in social settings, nearly paralyzed me for years. Rather than enjoy the company of those around me, I sadly spent my time focusing my will to avoid breaking into a cold sweat.

In addition, for reasons I didn't fully understand, my voice would fail me after eating, taking my characteristically authoritative voice to a loud whisper. Invariably, with my confidence shot, I would say something dumb, or was it because I said something dumb that my confidence was shot? It was getting hard to tell.

Looking back, it's all painfully clear to me. Things started to slide downhill when I started taking the acid reflux medications. I would later learn the headaches, apathy, and anxiety were common side effects of acid reflux medications. For many reasons, it was easy for me to miss the connection between the medication and its numerous side effects. A lot was changing for me during this time in my personal and work life, and I chalked it up to the stress of managing increasing responsibility.

Ultimately, what began as a little indigestion and irritation, ended in a full onslaught of my senses, my self-worth, and my outlook on life. Over a 15 year period, I went through the phases of occasional indigestion, to acid reflux, to GERD, and then full on silent reflux. I contemplated surgery early on and again many years later when I was diagnosed with a hiatal hernia. Thankfully, I ruled it out as within six months of my symptoms growing completely out of control, I found my cure.

Introduction

As you may have discovered, there is endless information online concerning reflux, its diagnoses, management, and treatment. This torrent of information comes in the form of diets, cookbooks, exercises, acupuncture, chiropractics, supplements, tips & tricks, hacks, etc...

Many of the so-called health influencers do not have personal experience dealing with reflux and therefore are unable to help you separate the facts from the fiction. Most, I would assume, are well intentioned but without medical or personal experience they have to SWAG (make Scientific Wild A** Guesses). Ultimately, however, these SWAGs do not hold water or stomach contents for that matter! As a result, their recommendations are further propagation of bad advice which leads to inconsistencies and mixed results. Of course, the worst among them are just trying to make a quick buck.

In contrast, I have personally applied every approach in this book. All of the conclusions and recommendations are rooted in science and discussed in simple terms. The underlying research is referenced throughout the book, should you be interested in further or deeper study. This is for all my fellow nerds out there.

This book is for sufferers of acid reflux, GERD, silent reflux (LPR), and its many related forms. In it, I will cover a wide range of topics designed to provide you with a holistic understanding of the disease, its history, prevalence, symptoms, diagnostics, triggers, root causes, and treatments.

The concepts enclosed in this book will no-doubt prompt you to re-evaluate what you thought you knew about reflux. Your learning doesn't have to end with the information included in this book. Get access to new content by joining my mailing list at:

TheAcidRefluxGuy.com/BookMailingList

or following me at:

TheAcidRefluxGuy.com/Instagram
TheAcidRefluxGuy.com/Pinterest
TheAcidRefluxGuy.com/YouTube
TheAcidRefluxGuy.com/Twitter

Armed with this knowledge and the practical steps that I took, I pray you will be able to join me and the many who have found relief, via TheAcidRefluxGuy.com, in beating this terrible disease!

Chapter 1

Acid Reflux Disease

I can tell you the exact moment that my reflux symptoms escalated into full-fledged silent reflux. It was near the end of the day, and I grabbed a handful of wint-o-green lifesavers, a growing habit after my administrative assistant learned that they were my favorite. After crunching down on the first few, I noticed my nose started to drip backwards into my throat. I thought that I was coming down with a cold, but something told me it was related to the candy that I had obsessively been devouring. The mucus did not persist, so I chalked it up to a 24-hour bug. After a two week break from the candies, I went for them again. This time, after that familiar mucus formed, it stayed with and tormented me until I found my cure.

* * *

The Many Faces of Acid Reflux

Acid Reflux has a long list of potential symptoms that can combine in seemingly countless combinations. As a result, there are many named reflux diseases, each with their own categorization of side effects. Most often, symptoms are grouped under three common labels:

- Acid Reflux
- Gastroesophageal Reflux Disease (GERD)
- Laryngopharyngeal Reflux (LPR / Silent Reflux)

It is important to clearly define a few terms. To that end, let's start with *acid reflux*. Typically, this term is used as a broad brush to refer to all forms of reflux diseases, regardless of the severity, intensity, or the expression of symptoms. Recognizing this term is overloaded, I will define it more precisely for the purposes of this text.

Acid Reflux

In the simplest terms, acid reflux is a disorder whereby stomach contents are able to flow backwards out of the stomach into the throat (esophagus). Oftentimes, acid reflux is accompanied by one or more of the following symptoms:

- Burning sensation in the chest (known as heartburn)
- Gas and bloating
- Sour taste
- Coughing
- Regurgitation of stomach contents

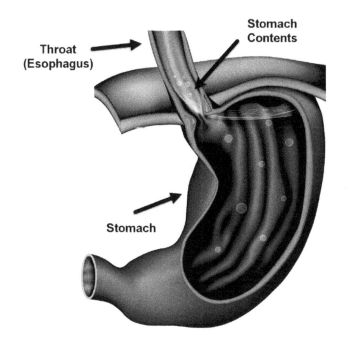

Figure 1

Generally speaking, these symptoms occur on an infrequent basis. For that reason, acid reflux is seemingly considered by the medical profession as more of a nuisance than a truly impactful disease. Of course, those of us on the other side of that statement beg to differ! As you progress further in this text, you will see that the ostensibly cavalier approach to the disease has lasting ramifications for sufferers.

Gastroesophageal Reflux Disease (GERD)

Next, we have Gastroesophageal Reflux Disease or GERD for short. GERD includes all the symptoms of acid reflux and is defined as acid reflux that occurs a minimum of two times per week or with increased severity. It comes with an additional set of symptoms such as:

- Difficulty swallowing
- Feeling of a lump in your throat
- Hoarseness
- Chronic coughing
- Throat clearing
- Bad breath
- Productive belching
- Throat inflammation
- Nausea
- Sleep issues

Laryngopharyngeal Reflux (LPR / Silent Reflux)

Last, but certainly not least, there is Laryngopharyngeal Reflux (LPR), whose symptoms were formally categorized in the 1970's. This little devil has a nasty habit of masquerading as other respiratory and ear-nose-throat disorders. For this reason it is often misdiagnosed as asthma, allergies, sinusitis, sleep apnea, etc. In fact, according to the National Library of Medicine 50 to 78% of the population with voice complaints and 91% of voice disorders can be attributed to LPR (Lechein, "Impact of LPR").

Additionally, LPR can be expressed without heartburn, the classic symptom of acid reflux and GERD. This is why it has earned the name silent reflux. This form of reflux brings with it a whole host of additional potential complications including:

- Hoarseness
- Chronic cough
- Post nasal drip
- Trouble breathing
- Excessive mucus
- Inflammation of the ear, nose, throat, and mouth

Relationship Between Acid Reflux, GERD, and Silent Reflux

As with GERD, silent reflux symptoms can be additive to acid reflux or GERD symptoms. In reality, each of the three diseases are a convenient categorization of common symptoms, but the symptoms are by no means mutually exclusive of each other. That means you may experience one or more of the symptoms listed across any of the three groups.

Looking back on my fifteen years with reflux, I can clearly see the causal factors that initiated my transition from acid reflux to GERD and GERD to silent reflux. These transitions were distinct, sudden, and very clearly linked to risk factors that I unwittingly triggered. That said, all along I had the persistent cough, hoarseness, excessive throat clearing which are characteristic of silent reflux, just less severe. It's as though all the ingredients were present and just waiting for the oven to hit the right temperature.

Long Term Effects of Acid Reflux

It is common knowledge now that acid reflux medications lead to several deficiencies including magnesium, calcium, and vitamin B12. In 2010, studies revealed increased risk of hip, wrist, and spine fracture when PPIs are taken more than once daily for more than a year. Subsequently, the United States Food and Drug Administration (FDA) required manufacturers to add a warning label to their products. In 2011, they issued a warning that long term use could lead to low magnesium or hypomagnesemia.

For example, studies have shown that taking PPIs for more than 2 years comes with a 65% increased likelihood of vitamin B12 deficiency. Similarly, a meta-analysis of more than 100,000 patients found a 43% increased risk of magnesium deficiency *(Srinutta, "PPI and Hypomagnesemia")*. Understanding the important function of these vitamins, it's not surprising that there is a 41% increased risk of bone fracture *(Nassar, "PPI Use and Fracture Risk")* and 44% increased risk of dementia *(Solan, "Can Heartburn Drug Cause Cognitive Problems")*. Below is a selection of the most common side effects of these vitamin deficiencies. For reference, I have bolded the symptoms that I personally dealt with:

- Weakness, **tiredness,** or lightheadedness
- Heart palpitations and shortness of breath
- Pale skin
- **A smooth tongue**
- Constipation, diarrhea, loss of appetite, or gas
- Nerve problems like numbness, **muscle weakness**, and problems walking
- **Vision loss**
- Mental problems like **depression, memory loss, or behavioral changes**
- Muscle Problems (aches, cramps, spasms, numbness, **tingling in hands**, arms, feet, legs and **around the mouth**)
- **Extreme fatigue**
- Nail and skin symptoms (itch, inflammation, psoriasis)
- Osteopenia and osteoporosis (low bone density)
- Painful PMS
- Dental problems
- Nausea
- Loss of appetite
- **Anxiety**

If you experience any of these symptoms, you may be deficient.

How Acid Reflux Affects Quality of Life

In the below graph, I have charted my personal experience with reflux symptoms using the Global Overall Symptom scale. The assessment provides an objective method to measure the severity of symptoms across 25 questions and 5 quality of life dimensions including emotional distress, sleep disturbance, food/drink problems, physical/social functioning and vitality *(Veldhuyzen van Zanten, "Validation of a 7-point")*. These are measured on a scale of ratings from 1 = no problem to 7 = very severe problem. In this case, I assessed myself three times, one for each phase of my disease.

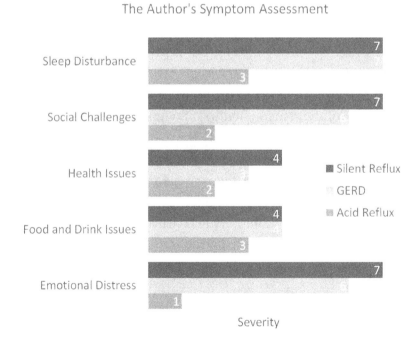

Figure 2

Quality of Life categories:

- Sleep Disturbance - breathing difficulty, overheating, choking, coughing, muscle spasms
- Social Challenges - hoarseness, clearing throat, coughing, belching, limitations of daily activities
- Health Issues - chest pain, constipation, excess mucus / post nasal drip, gastric pain, diarrhea, globus, difficulty swallowing, breathing difficulties, choking episodes, use of unprescribed medication
- Food and Drink Issues - regurgitation, indigestion, eating problems
- Emotional Distress - anxiety, apathy, behavioral changes

Global Overall Symptom (GOS) Scale:

- 1 - No problem
- 2 - Minimal problem (can be easily ignored without effort)
- 3 - Mild problem (can be ignored with effort)
- 4 - Moderate problem (cannot be ignored but does not influence my daily activities)
- 5 - Moderately severe problem (cannot be ignored and occasionally limits my daily activities)
- 6 - Severe problem (cannot be ignored and often limits my concentration on daily activities)
- 7 - Very severe problem (cannot be ignored and markedly limits my daily activities and often requires rest)

For me, emotional distress, social challenges, and sleep disturbance were the more devastating aspects of my disease. Many who contact me seem to struggle most with food/drink, health issues, and the associated emotional distress.

Summary

In this chapter, we have covered the three primary categorizations of acid reflux symptoms (acid reflux, GERD, and silent reflux). Additionally, I explained that these symptoms actually combine in unique ways for each individual. It is important to note that while the expression of the various acid reflux diseases and symptoms can vary, the risk factors and root causes for the disease are actually quite consistent. We will explore both in greater detail in the chapters to come.

Chapter 2

Epidemiology

One of my first anxiety attacks happened early in my career, while I was in a staff meeting at work. My boss, presumably complementary, commented that I got up to speed on a new technology much faster than she would have expected. This embarrassed me slightly, which raised my body temperature enough to trigger my body to spontaneously go into full body sweats as if I just finished running a marathon. To add insult to injury, one of my colleagues locked eyes with me from across the table and mouthed "Wuss!" Years later, I learned that anxiety (and my full body sweat response) is one of the many fun side effects of acid reflux medications.

* * *

Global Impact

The term epidemiology refers to the branch of medicine that among other things, deals with the prevalence of disease and its contributing factors. So in this chapter we will spend a little time zooming out to look at the disease, its impact globally, and how that has changed over time.

To start with, it may surprise you to learn that acid reflux is actually the most widespread gastrointestinal disorder in the United States *(Richter, "Presentation and Epidemiology")*. It alone accounts for a whopping $20 billion of the total $142 billion spent on gastrointestinal diseases *(Thomas, "GERD: Facts, Statistics")*. More than $10 billion of that is spent on the various acid reflux medications *(Young, "Holiday Meals Don't Have to Burn")*.

Furthermore, the disease led to a staggering 4.7 million hospital admissions in 2010, which is up from over 1 million just twelve years earlier in 1998 *(Thomas, "GERD: Facts, Statistics")*. In fact, the occurrence of GERD is reported to have increased more than 50% globally, over the last decade *(Boyles, "Study: Acid Reflux on the Rise")*. These statistics highlight the ever increasing prevalence and severity of the disease.

With growth like that, it's not surprising that the National Cancer Institute shares that esophageal (throat) cancer is the fastest growing cancer across the United States, having increased 850% since 1975, with mortality increasing sevenfold *(The Voice Institute, "Silent Laryngopharyngeal Reflux (LPR)")*.

Looking at the below map, you can see estimated global distribution of the disease *(Dr. Guarner et. al., "Map of Digestive Disorders")*. Note the wide ranges across regions. This is due to cultural influences, timing, and variations in underlying studies such as thresholds for the duration and frequency of symptoms.

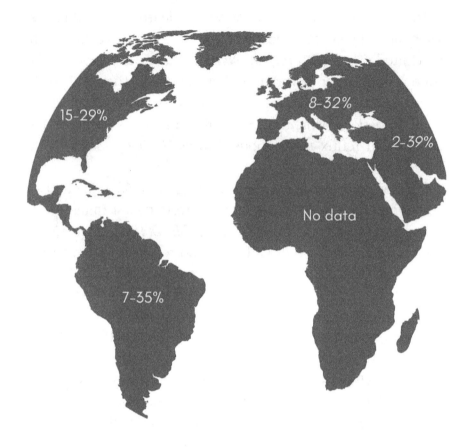

Figure 3

In total, this disease impacts an estimated 13% of the global population (nearly 1 in 8 people), albeit with significant geographic differences *(Richter, "Presentation and Epidemiology")*. It is not so much genetics as it is cultural influences that have a significant effect on the disease, its frequency and expressions because acid reflux is largely driven by environmental matters including lifestyle, disease, and medical factors.

Demographics

A wide scale study in the United States involving data from 54 million patients revealed that *(Yamasaki et al. "The Changing Epidemiology")*:

- 80% of acid reflux patients were caucasian
- Approximately 65% of GERD patients are women
- Most patients were considered obese (45%) or severely obese (31%)
- Most patients are greater than 70 years of age

Given these factors, you are at the greatest risk for developing acid reflux if you are a fair, full figured, seventy plus female. If this doesn't fit you, don't worry as averages can be misleading. I am actually precisely the opposite of this demographic as a young-ish (40), thin, black male! Also, I don't want you to confuse these traits as being causal for developing acid reflux. They are merely a correlation of the data and a gross simplification of the many factors that can lead to the development of the disease. As I mentioned earlier, this disease follows cultural norms, and therefore it should not be surprising to find that some cultures have a heavier occurrence of the disease.

For years we believed acid reflux was an elderly person's disease. However, recent studies looking at the last 10 years of data, have revealed that acid reflux is NOT exclusively limited to the elderly. In fact, the fastest increase in GERD diagnosis year over year is occurring in individuals in the range of 30-39 years of age *(Yamasaki et al. "The Changing Epidemiology")*.

Looking at symptoms of reflux, studies show that nearly 50% of patients report heartburn and regurgitation as their top symptoms followed by abdominal pain and bloating (Richter, "Presentation and Epidemiology"). Less common symptoms included: chest pain, hyper/acidic salivation, painful/trouble swallowing, burping, hiccups, nausea, and vomiting.

Least common of all, and the most resistant to medical / surgical treatments, are chronic cough, hoarseness, feeling of something in the throat (globus sensation), throat clearing, and respiratory issues. As you may have noticed, these "least common" symptoms are largely categorized under silent reflux. For reference, Dr. Koufman, who coined the phrase silent reflux, found that "10% of GERD patients who came to her clinic had LPR *(Kamani, "The Prevalence of L.P.R.")*.

A recent study conducted in the United Kingdom, found a strong correlation between silent reflux sufferers and medications, asthma, hiatal hernia, depression, lack of exercise, and Irritable Bowel Syndrome (IBS) *(Kamani, "The prevalence of L.P.R.")*. Causation was not established, meaning the study did not establish if these issues triggered silent reflux or if the reverse was true. This study also found that GERD sufferers are:

- **9 times more likely** to have silent reflux if they take reflux medications in combination with oral steroids, anti-inflammatories, arthritis, nerve blocking drugs, nitrates or heart disease drugs
- **7 times more likely** given a history of depression
- **4 times more likely** if they have Irritable Bowel Syndrome (IBS)
- **more likely** with higher Body-Mass-Index (BMI)
- **more likely** if between the age 18-40 vs +60

Triggers

A trigger is anything that escalates the symptoms of a disease that an individual already has. Typically, acid reflux sufferers are aware of food and drink that immediately trigger the escalation of their symptoms. That said, many are unaware that other food and drink items that they consume regularly are contributing to their discomfort and the escalation of symptoms. This, as it takes time for the offending food item to make its way through the digestive tract. Furthermore, some triggers lead to gut inflammation which can lead to longer term symptoms.

There are a wide array of foods and drinks that can trigger acid reflux so I cannot hope to cover them all in this book. Instead, the below chart covers triggers that are common to many reflux sufferers. It is important to note that eliminating these triggers from your diet will not eliminate reflux. At best, removal can help to address some of the variability and sharpness of symptoms.

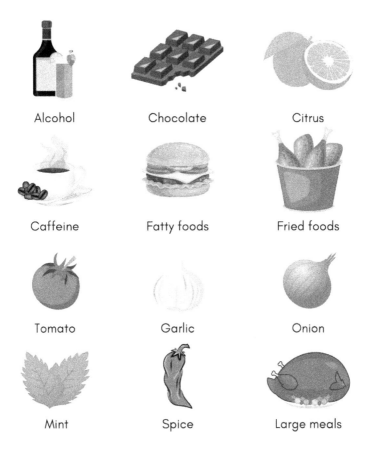

Figure 4

Risk Factors

In contrast to a trigger, which escalates an existing disease, a risk factor is anything that increases the likelihood or risk for a person to develop the disease or condition in the first place. That said, triggers and risk factors have one thing in common. Their removal often has limited to no effect on the underlying disease. It's a bit like getting an F on a test. Afterwards, it feels near impossible to get your average back up, no matter how many A's you subsequently achieve. In the future chapters, I cover reasons it is so challenging to recover once you have entered the reflux cycle.

As a conclusion to this chapter I will unpack each of the three risk factor categories that can lead to the onset of acid reflux. Each of these risk factors including lifestyle, disease, and medical can have one or more negative effects on digestive function. To help visualize this, I have grouped examples of each in the below diagram. In it, lifestyle factors are shown in normal text, disease factors are in bold, and medical factors are in bold and capital letters. The label 'CONTAIN' refers to effects on the body's ability to keep contents in the stomach until such time that it should be evacuated into the small intestines. The term 'DIGEST' refers to digestive balance and 'MOVE' refers to effective movement of food matter along the digestive tract.

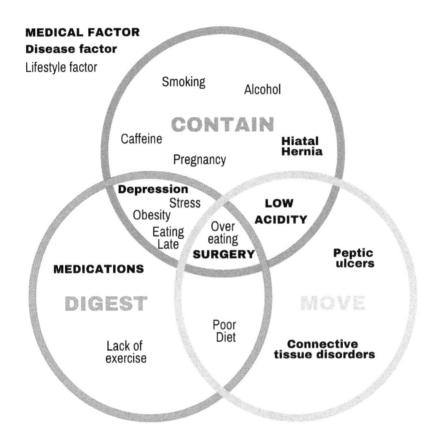

Figure 5

Lifestyle Factors

Quite interestingly, a majority of the *lifestyle* choices affect the body's ability to effectively contain stomach contents. Specifically, they affect lower esophageal sphincter and pyloric sphincter function. Under normal circumstances, these sphincters open and close to affect the flow of food through the digestive tract. The lower esophageal sphincter needs to remain closed to keep food contents out of the throat. The pyloric sphincter, which sits below the stomach, remains closed until the body is ready to release food into the intestines. If it remains closed too long then food sits on the stomach longer than it should, leading to indigestion.

It is common knowledge that exercise has a beneficial impact on metabolism and fitness. However, you may be surprised to learn that it also has a more immediate impact on digestive health and efficiency. This is achieved through a process called peristalsis, which moves food along the digestive tract through a series of involuntary yet coordinated muscle movements *(Chutkan, "The Microbiome Solution")*.

Lastly, the content of your diet has a direct effect on digestive health. The more narrow, processed, and high in sugar your food choices are, the more your digestive system is skewed to process these foods. This leads to harmful imbalances and side effects that negatively affect digestive efficiency. The effects are similar to that of long term depression or persistent stress, which I have classified as a disease factor.

Disease Factors

Providing an exhaustive list of *disease* factors is beyond the scope of this book. Instead, I have listed a few key factors including depression, hiatal hernia, peptic ulcers, and connective tissue disorders. To start, connective tissue disorders and ulcers can have detrimental effects on the effective passage of food through the digestive tract.

Studies have shown that when the body is under stress / depression the percentage of beneficial bacteria in your digestive tract declines and harmful pathogens quickly multiply to take their place (Madison, "Stress, depression, diet"). This imbalance is known as dysbiosis, which refers to a microbial imbalance in the body.

Medical Factors

Many times people struggle to identify risk factors that contributed to their acid reflux. However, that is not often the case for those who develop reflux as a side effect of a *medical* procedure or medication. In these cases, onset is sudden and more easily correlated to a life changing event. It's not surprising that acid reflux is the most prevalent outpatient gastrointestinal diagnosis. This, as precursors include a very long list of common medications including those for asthma, blood pressure, depression, sedatives, antidepressants, narcotics, tranquilizers, antibiotics, etc.

Note that the risk factors on the prior chart do not represent one-time events, rather they are persistent factors that over time can lead to reduced digestive function. As you can see there are several risk factors that affect two or more digestive functions. For instance, over-eating can have adverse effects along each dimension, especially when the diet has low food diversity and the food is high fat / sugar. If this describes your diet, you are not alone. In fact, according to FullScript.com the "Standard American Diet consists of ultra-processed foods, added sugar, fat, and sodium. Added sugars account for 13% of the average American's total caloric intake each day *(Dan, "The Standard American Diet")*." In the next chapter, I will explore the connection between these risk factors and the underlying root causes of reflux.

Summary

Acid reflux disease is quite prevalent globally. Studies have correlated many physical characteristics that exist across its wide base of sufferers. That said, many of these seemingly causal factors do not guarantee the presence of the disease so much as they often accompany it. However, it is quite clear that certain lifestyles, diseases, and medical factors increase the likelihood of pushing an individual into the reflux cycle. In the subsequent chapters, we will look at the most common root causes behind the onset and escalation of this disease.

Chapter 3

Diagnostic Tools

I often went through 2-3 king sized bottles of antacids per month. They were my go-to in the middle of the night, when I woke with a mouth full of stomach acid and mucus. I also carried them in my bag for work, bag for the gym, and was sure to pack copious amounts for business trips. Any increase in my body temperature or change to the angle of my sleep often left me in poor shape.

* * *

My Experience with Diagnostics

Earlier, I shared my experiences with acid reflux and how its symptoms progressed in frequency and intensity over a 15 year period. This is a pattern that I have seen play out as I study the disease and its epidemiology, and as I speak to hundreds of individuals who have contacted me via TheAcidRefluxGuy.com.

Despite the long term physical and psychological ramifications of acid reflux, many doctors seem to quickly triage and prescribe medications as they might a simple viral or bacterial infection. My first visit to my primary care physician went like this: The physician listened to a couple minutes of symptoms, asked me a few questions, asked me to stick out my tongue, and say ahh... then prescribed 10mg of Prilosec.

Done! No diagnostics, no tests to determine the nature of my disease, and no referral to a specialist. I didn't know to ask for any of these things. I simply trusted that the doctor understood my condition and provided me with the right remedy. I actually left the doctor believing the prescription would heal my reflux. However, after a couple weeks, I found that I couldn't stop taking the medicines, and I was back at the doctor's office looking for a renewed prescription.

In the years to follow, doctors would double my dose of prescription PPIs two times, from 10mg to 40mg per day, due to escalating symptoms. It was around the seven year mark that my doctor ordered my very first diagnostic, an Esophagogastroduodenoscopy (EGD). After seven years of dealing with the increasingly severe symptoms of acid reflux, I would finally learn from the EGD that I have a hiatal hernia.

During the procedure, the doctor also took a tissue sample from my stomach as prolonged use of prescription reflux medication often causes the development of polyps which can turn cancerous. Thankfully, these came back negative and as I write this now, 8 years later, I have not done a follow up test. I pray that I still remain cancer free, but the reality remains a daunting possibility in my future. I have enclosed my EGD results below. In it, you can see my stomach polyps [image reference #1] and my bulbous lower esophageal sphincter / hiatal hernia [image reference #6].

Endoscopy

Patient Name:	Daniels, Don J.	**Procedure Date:**	9/23/2013 10:42 AM
MRN:		**Date of Birth:**	
Age:	33	**Gender:**	Male
Note Status:	Finalized	**Attending MD:**	

Procedure: Upper GI endoscopy
Indications: Heartburn
Providers:

Referring MD:
Medicines: Monitored Anesthesia Care
Complications: No immediate complications.

Procedure: After obtaining informed consent, the endoscope was passed under direct vision. Throughout the procedure, the patient's blood pressure, pulse, and oxygen saturations were monitored continuously. The GIF Q160 025 was introduced through the mouth, and advanced to the second part of duodenum. The upper GI endoscopy was accomplished without difficulty. The patient tolerated the procedure well.

Upper Gastrointestinal Tract

Findings:

The examined esophagus was normal. Biopsies were taken with a cold forceps for histology.

Multiple 5 to 9 mm pedunculated and sessile polyps with no stigmata of recent bleeding were found in the gastric body. The polyp was removed with a cold biopsy forceps. Resection and retrieval were complete.

Localized mild inflammation characterized by congestion (edema) was found in the gastric antrum. Biopsies were taken with a cold forceps for histology.

The examined duodenum was normal.

Add'l Images:

1 Gastric Body   2 Duodenal Bulb   3 2nd Portion of the Duodenum   4 Gastric Body

Figure 6

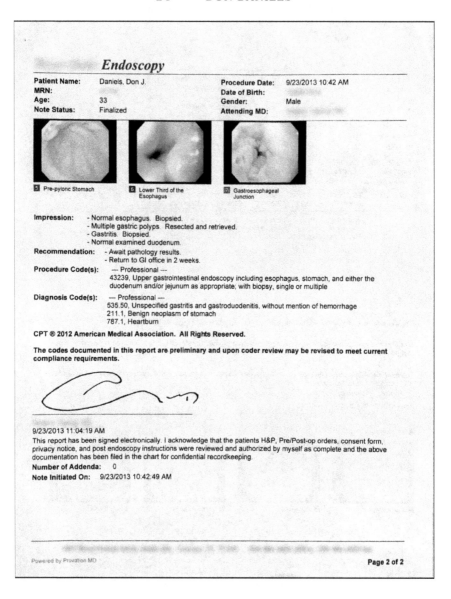

Endoscopy

Patient Name:	Daniels, Don J.	**Procedure Date:**	9/23/2013 10:42 AM
MRN:		**Date of Birth:**	
Age:	33	**Gender:**	Male
Note Status:	Finalized	**Attending MD:**	

5 Pre-pylonc Stomach   6 Lower Third of the Esophagus   7 Gastroesophageal Junction

Impression: - Normal esophagus. Biopsied.
- Multiple gastric polyps. Resected and retrieved.
- Gastritis. Biopsied.
- Normal examined duodenum.

Recommendation: - Await pathology results.
- Return to GI office in 2 weeks.

Procedure Code(s): --- Professional ---
43239, Upper gastrointestinal endoscopy including esophagus, stomach, and either the duodenum and/or jejunum as appropriate; with biopsy, single or multiple

Diagnosis Code(s): --- Professional ---
535.50, Unspecified gastritis and gastroduodenitis, without mention of hemorrhage
211.1, Benign neoplasm of stomach
787.1, Heartburn

CPT ® 2012 American Medical Association. All Rights Reserved.

The codes documented in this report are preliminary and upon coder review may be revised to meet current compliance requirements.

9/23/2013 11:04:19 AM
This report has been signed electronically. I acknowledge that the patients H&P, Pre/Post-op orders, consent form, privacy notice, and post endoscopy instructions were reviewed and authorized by myself as complete and the above documentation has been filed in the chart for confidential recordkeeping.
Number of Addenda: 0
Note Initiated On: 9/23/2013 10:42:49 AM

Powered by Provation MD   Page 2 of 2

Figure 7

Fast forward another seven years, my reflux had escalated to full-fledged silent reflux. At this point, my reflux would not respond to a third doubling my prescription (to 80mg). As a result, my doctor ordered my second and third diagnostic tests, a sleep apnea, and Helicobacter pylori (H. pylori) test. As you may have experienced, doctors often miss-attribute silent reflux to a wide array breathing disorders. In my case this was sleep apnea. However, to my increasing dismay, both tests turned up negative.

In the chart below, you can see the progression of my reflux disease and where critical lifestyle changes escalated my symptoms. There were medical factors as well which we will explore later.

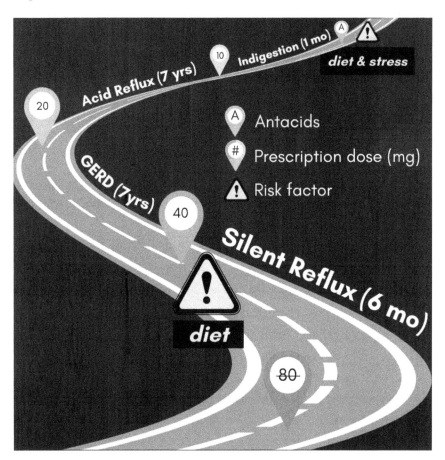

Figure 8

To put this in perspective, over fifteen years, I only received three diagnostic tests to determine the nature of my increasingly severe reflux disease. I feel that more diagnostics could have been done proactively vs reactively as a means to perform a thorough situational analysis. In my mind, the first step to treatment should be a complete understanding of the root causes of the condition. Something we will focus heavily on in this text.

Acid Reflux Diagnostics

All this being said, I do want to provide a quick overview of the key diagnostic tools that are available so you are able to have an informed discussion with your medical provider and can hopefully fast track the diagnosis of your condition. Below, I have compiled a list of relevant and available diagnostics *(WebMD, "Diagnosing Acid Reflux Disease")* and *(US National Library of Medicine, "Helicobacter Pylori")*.

- Barium Swallow Radiograph - After swallowing a barium solution an x-ray machine scans for damage to your esophagus (inner throat).
- Esophagogastroduodenoscopy (EGD) - A small tube with a camera is inserted, enabling visual inspection of your esophagus and stomach. The procedure is done under local or general anesthesia (numbing or sleeping agent to eliminate discomfort).
- Biopsy - A tissue sample is extracted from the inner lining of your stomach so it can be scanned for signs of cancer. This test can be done in conjunction with the EGD procedure.
- Esophageal Manometry - A small tube inserted through your nose to the lower region of your esophagus. This is used to record muscle contractions and verify function of your lower esophageal sphincter (LES), your primary anti-reflux barrier.
- Esophageal Impedance Monitoring - Uses a small tube to measure flow of liquids through your esophagus to de-

termine how effectively your body moves food through your esophagus to your stomach.

- pH Monitoring - A small tube with a pH (measure of acidity) sensor is passed through your nose to your esophagus for 24 hours. This test measures the presence of acids over that period.
- Helicobacter pylori (H. pylori) Test - Analyzes blood, stool, or breath to identify a bacterial infection known to trigger reflux symptoms.
- Heidelberg Test – The patient swallows a small transceiver which relays a continuous measurement of stomach pH to a computer. After swallowing a sodium bicarbonate solution, the test measures the time it takes for stomach acidity to return to normal. Based on this the patient is diagnosed as having low (hypochlorhydria), no (achlorhydria), or high stomach acid (hypochlorhydria).
- Gut Test – A stool sample is analyzed to determine the presence and diversity of certain species of microorganisms. For a home gut test kit, see TheAcidRefluxGuy.com/Resources.

Summary

Hopefully, after speaking with your doctor about these diagnostics, you can gain additional clarity into your condition. That said, I want to make a special note regarding silent reflux as it is particularly difficult for doctors to diagnose. This is because it's fairly uncommon and its symptoms are non-distinct from those of infection, strained voice, smoking, heavy drinking, allergies, asthma, and other respiratory ailments.

Furthermore, there are no diagnostic tests to definitively diagnose silent reflux as distinct from GERD or acid reflux. That said, there is a quiz called the Reflux Symptom Index that can be taken to determine the likelihood that you have silent reflux. To take this quiz for yourself, go to: TheAcidRefluxGuy.com/SilentRefluxQuiz.

Even specialists, such as Ear-Nose-Throat (ENT) doctors ostensibly receive little specific training on silent reflux in their residency programs and continuing education. In an, admittedly small, survey of fifty one doctors, 45% were familiar with LPR, and 16% were familiar with the Reflux Symptom Index *(Chorti, "Knowledge of Primary Care Doctors")*. This bears out in the experiences that individuals have relayed to me and, perhaps, with your own experience.

As such, you may need to help your doctor make the connection by introducing the idea and correlating your symptoms to the more well-known symptoms of acid reflux and GERD. Part of the problem, it seems, is that no medical specialists claim LPR as their domain. ENTs are referred most often, but if you can get a referral, your best bet might be with a Gastroenterologist. Better yet, would be a doctor who specializes in Functional Medicine.

As I have said before, I was diagnosed (by way of EGD) with a hiatal hernia, which is an impairment of the lower esophageal sphincter, and part of a muscle ring in your throat that forms your primary anti-reflux barrier. Unfortunately, with this information, I was resigned to the fact that I would deal with reflux for the rest of my life. Thankfully, this was simply not true! What I didn't know then, but, I know now, is that many people have hiatal hernias, but no reflux. One does not guarantee the other!

Chapter 4

Medical Treatments

"I have somebody I want you to meet." Those words came to strike terror into my heart as my social anxiety grew. Invariably, after church concluded, my wife would have some person she wanted me to build a connection with. This, inevitably, meant I would need to pass dozens of friendly faces who would want to greet me, on the complete other side of our large church building, just to meet the one person my wife actually had in mind for me to meet. A terrifying proposition for one who's ability to concentrate on discussions and fully articulate thoughts had been waning. Besides, it took all my energy to avoid breaking into a sweat.

* * *

History of Acid Reflux Treatments

As far back as the first century, chewing chalks, green tea, magnesia, and food-grade charcoals, were common remedies to indigestion *(Modlin. "Historical perspectives")*. It may surprise you, but we're still chewing chalk as a primary means to manage reflux. This is because chalk (calcium carbonate) is the active ingredient in Tums, Alka-Seltzer, Mylanta, and other over the counter antacids. The truth is very little has changed in 1,000 years, despite all our advances in technology and the fact that acid reflux is now one of the most globally widespread medical conditions.

For most of human history, we did not fully understand concepts of stomach acid and digestion. It wasn't until the early 1800's, that a freak accident created the perfect conditions to document the digestive process. A military surgeon, named William Beaumont, received a patient who was accidentally struck in the stomach with shotgun pellets when a loaded shotgun discharged. Beaumont performed surgery, saving the patient's life, but amazingly the wound never closed. With the cooperation of his patient, Beaumont began conducting experiments by tying food to a string and inserting it into the stomach through the hole! Every so often, he would pull the food out to observe and record the state of digestion. This cornerstone study served as foundational in our understanding of stomach acid, and the part it plays in digestion.

By the early 20th century, reflux mitigation tactics shifted to avoiding trigger foods, wearing loose clothing, weight loss, and aggressive acid neutralization. The diet based techniques found mixed success as most require catching the disease early or long term discipline. Furthermore, they largely offer symptom mitigation, not healing. Some of the more aggressive approaches such as acid neutralization and alkali diets/drinks resulted in dangerous syndromes affecting bone density, causing organ failure, neurological and neuromuscular dysfunctions *(Modlin. "Historical Perspectives")*.

Surgical Procedures

Attempts to provide longer term remedies led to the rise of novel surgical techniques. The Nissen Fundoplication, for instance, was one such technique that boasts more than 100,000 surgeries per year since the 1990s. Sadly, while it reports up to a 90% success rate, studies have shown up to 27% failure rate over 10 years.

A similar percentage suffer post-surgical complications such as the inability to burp (61%) or suffering persistent flatulence (91%), inability to vomit (31%), and bloating (72%) *(Kellokumpu, "QoL Following Laparoscopic Nissen")*. Reviews of a dozen such alternative surgical procedures show similarly mixed results. Not surprisingly, I have had a number of people contact me, having relapsed post-surgery.

Medications

As of the writing of this book, omeprazole, a prescription reflux medication, is the #7 most prescribed medicine in the United States behind popular thyroid, blood pressure, choles-terol, and diabetes medications *(Lewis, "The Top 50 Drugs")*.

Given this and the $10 billion spent on similar medications, you would think that the prevalence of acid reflux diseases would be in decline. However, our review of epidemiology showed precisely the opposite. As we have covered prior, since their advent in the 1970's, the prevalence of acid reflux dis-eases has increased at an alarming rate. In fact, Adenocarci-noma, a cancer closely linked with heartburn has become the fastest growing cancer and is now the 7th leading cause of death in men *(Eldridge, "Top 10 Cancers Causing Death")*.

Do you find it strange that acid reflux disease has increased in frequency and severity since the advent of these drugs? Could there be a causal relationship between the use of these drugs and the increasing severity? Hold that thought as we will explore this further in future chapters.

For now, let's cover the four categories of reflux medica-tions: Antacids, H2 Receptor Blockers (H2 Blockers), Proton Pump Inhibitors (PPIs), and Prokinetic agents (Pro-kinetics). It is important to understand these medications and how they affect your body.

Antacids

I often consider antacids to be the gateway drug of acid reflux. They offer a "quick fix," they taste like candy, and they're Over the Counter (OTC) so you can get them on any street corner. The marketing and "social proof" of antacids are so strong that people pick them up on a whim at the first onset of irritation. I took Pepto Bismol and Tums for a while before moving on to the hard stuff.

Knowing prescriptions aren't a complete solution, doctors often send their patients home with a prescription for acid reflux medications and a recommendation to grab some antacids to manage flair ups. They come in several forms including chewables, dissolvable tablets, and liquids. They also come in many different formulations including aluminum, calcium carbonate, sodium bicarbonate, and magnesium oxide *(Ogbru, "Antacids")*. The variety enables combinations with other drugs, ability to avoid allergies, and offers differences in responsiveness and duration.

One common theme among the first three categories of acid reflux medications we cover (antacids, H2 blockers, and PPIs) is that they each focus on suppressing, neutralizing, or blocking the production of stomach acids. Antacids focus on reducing the acidity of stomach acid by neutralizing it. To understand this, we first need to understand how stomach acid is measured using the pH scale.

The pH scale measures the potency of an acid or base and is expressed as a number from 1 – 14 (though technically, this scale is open ended and values can range from 0 to +14 plus). Water, for instance, is neither an acid nor a base and it sits in the middle of this scale with a 7 pH. Acids, on the other hand, have a low pH number ranging from 1 to slightly less than 7, whereas a base has high pH ranging from slightly more than 7 to 14 *(Fookes, "Antacids").*

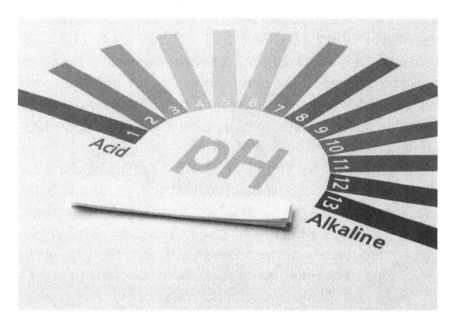

Figure 9

Under normal conditions, stomach acid is in the range of 1-3 pH, so it is HIGHLY acidic. Antacids, a base (or alkaline) substance, are in the 9-10 pH range. As you would expect, the more antacids you consume, the more your stomach acid moves towards a more neutral pH of 7 (like water). In fact, there is an antacid rating scale called the Antacid's Neutral-izing Capacity (ANC) that measures the effectiveness of an antacid ability to neutralize stomach acid to a pH of 3.5-4 *(Ogbru, "Antacids").* Antacids have a near immediate effect on symptoms by quickly neutralizing acid from sensitive areas of the body. However, as you might imagine, lower acidity also re-duces the effectiveness of your stomach acid when digesting food.

H2 (Histamine-2) Blockers

I still remember my first doctor's visit for acid reflux, now more than 15 years ago. They wanted to prescribe Zantac (Ranitidine), a popular H2 blocker that was later withdrawn from the market by the Food and Drug Administration (FDA), due to concentrations of NDMA, a known carcinogen linked to prostate, esophageal and other cancers. Thankfully, I had tried it prior, and found that it had no effect on my reflux symptoms. Instead, they prescribed a proton pump inhibitor, which I took dutifully for the next 15 years.

Histamine H2-Receptor Antagonists, or H2 Blockers for short, work by decreasing acid production in the stomach lining. Normally, cells in your stomach lining release histamines, which stimulates acid-producing cells. The drugs are absorbed quickly and are shown to decrease acid secretions by up to 70% for up to 24-hours *(Kerr, "H2 Receptor Blockers")*.

You can get H2 blockers in a wide variety of forms including tablets, liquids, capsules, and as injections. There are four types including Famotidine, Cimetidine, Ranitidine, and Nazatidine *(AboutGERD.org, "H2 Blockers")*. These are better known in their branded forms including Pepcid, Tagamet, Zantac, etc. H2 Blockers are generally less effective at reducing the severity of symptoms as compared to their more potent cousins, the Proton Pump Inhibitors.

Proton Pump Inhibitors (PPIs)

According to the National Institutes of Health, PPIs account for 95% of acid-suppressing drugs. *(Ka Seng Thong, "PPI and Fracture Risk")*. Given the prevalence, I could have written about PPIs first as they are the mainstay of the mainstream acid reflux treatment plan. But, I intentionally went from antacids to H2 Blockers to PPIs as a way to show the progression in potency as well as to mirror the common path that acid reflux sufferers take as their disease progresses. We have not discussed root causes yet or the reasons for the progression; however, I expect you may have experienced this first hand.

PPIs are fairly similar to H2 Blockers in that they ultimately block the production of stomach acids. The difference, however, is in the method. After PPIs absorb into the blood, they effectively stop the stomach's protein pump from expressing acid into the stomach, hence their name.

As opposed to Antacids, which have an immediate effect, or H2's which can absorb and take limited effect within hours, PPIs accumulate over the course of days. The effects are longer term and the drug is designed to be taken over time at regular intervals.

Quite interestingly, studies have shown they offer relief to 78-92% of patients when taken once daily. However, this is merely mitigation (not healing) as recurrence of symptoms occurs at a rate of 75-90% of patients who stop taking them *(Lemperle, "G.E.R.D")*. I expect you have experienced this rebound yourself. When I forgot to take my medicine, I devolved into a coughing hacking mess within an hour or two of my mistake.

More times than I would like to admit, I had to stop doing what I was doing to run to the corner pharmacy and pick up an OTC that could help resume managing my symptoms. I could barely make it through the day if I did not have them in my system. Did that make me a junkie?

I should also say that PPIs alone were never enough to manage my symptoms. I ate antacids by the fistful, especially at night when my indigestion and regurgitation symptoms seemed to flair the worst. This seems to be quite common across reflux sufferers as evidenced in studies and my experiences working with individuals who visit my site.

Prokinetic Agents

There is a fourth category of acid reflux medication called prokinetics. I included it here for completeness, as it is only prescribed in severe cases of acid reflux disease due to potentially serious side effects. In her book "Prokinetics and Acid Reflux," Patricia Raymond shares that with regards to potency, prokinetics fall between H2 blockers and PPIs. Additionally, the prokinetic agent works quite differently as compared to its medicinal brethren and is most often paired up with H2 blockers or PPIs. The drugs don't stay in the bloodstream long and are consequently taken 2-4 times a day before meals and bedtime *(Raymond, "Prokinetics and Acid Reflux")*.

Prokinetics focus on improving lower esophageal sphincter (LES) function as well as movement of food through the digestive tract. The drug reportedly increases the pressure exerted by the LES, thereby better managing reflux. Additionally, they strengthen the muscular walls of your digestive tract, prompting foods to move through your digestive system efficiently, leading to less indigestion.

I do not have first-hand experience with prokinetics, however my research indicates they can be effective enough when used in combination with the other medications to effectively mitigate the symptoms of reflux. That said, they are not widely prescribed due to the wide range of bizarre and severe side effects, from slurred speech to inappropriate milk release from the breasts even in men.

Summary

Each of the four medications we have reviewed have short term perceived benefits in managing acid reflux symptoms. As is typical, medications have positives and negatives that need to be considered when evaluating treatment options.

The Federal Drug Administration advises that any of these medications should not be taken for more than 14 days. However, some doctors will extend this to 6-8 weeks. These drugs are not intended for long term use. They are not a cure as they do little more than manage symptoms, albeit poorly... So you might ask what are they good for?

In my opinion, due to the many serious side effects their use should really be limited to healing ulcers and inflammatory conditions such as gastritis or esophagitis. In this case, the medications can be used to reduce and restrict acidity and allow time for ulcers and gastrointestinal inflammation to heal. Beyond this, my experience is that they do far more damage than they do good.

Chapter 5

Underlying Root Causes

My wife affectionately referred to them as "pre-naps." You know the nap you take before you go to bed. Invariably, by Thursday of each week I was so utterly exhausted from poor sleep and the work week that I fell asleep in a sitting position on the couch. My attempt to "rest my eyes" turned into a full-fledged slumber fest. The problem was, my reflux demanded that I sleep on my stomach as any other position resulted in a throat and mouth full of stomach acid and mucus. The nap felt good, but I often spent the next fifteen minutes coughing, gagging, and popping antacids to clear my throat.

* * *

Having reviewed the common risk factors (lifestyle, disease, and medical), we understand some of the precursors to reflux disease. With this foundation we can look at the actual mechanisms in the body that can get out of balance and enable the disease to manifest.

You saw earlier in this text that an estimated 13% of the global population suffer from acid reflux. So why is it that the other 87% of people do not? We know by reading through the risk factors that quite a number of people have lifestyles where one or more risks are present, yet they do not have acid reflux.

This is because the body is incredibly resilient, able to self-heal, and rebalance to resolve a wide array of issues. In addition, the body is equipped with five anti-reflux mechanisms. When functioning as designed, three of these mechanisms automatically prevent reflux from occurring in the base case. If, however, stomach contents do escape, the other two quickly kick in to neutralize and mitigate any potential damage. Let's explore each of these rebalance and anti-reflux mechanisms through the remainder of this chapter.

Lower Esophageal Sphincter, Diaphragmatic Sphincter, and Pyloric Sphincter

Your body's primary anti-reflux barrier is a type of muscle called a sphincter. A sphincter is a highly specialized type of muscle that is organized in a ring and can be used to allow or restrict passage of fluids and materials through your body.

You are probably most familiar with three that are under your conscious control, namely the anal sphincter (allows you to poop), urethral sphincter (allows you to pee), and the upper esophageal sphincter (allows you to swallow). At will, you are able to contract and relax these muscles to allow the passage of food and drink into and out of your body.

The sphincter is a common design pattern that is reused throughout the human body. In fact, there are more than 60 types of sphincters, including the millions of precapillary sphincters that control blood flow through your blood vessels. The vast majority of these sphincters are under the control of your central nervous system. That's a good thing, because it would be a lot to remember and coordinate on a daily basis.

Similarly, there are two sphincters in your esophagus that are responsible for opening and closing the junction between your stomach and throat. These two muscles, the Lower Esophageal Sphincter (LES) and diaphragmatic sphincters are responsible for keeping your stomach contents in your stomach. These muscles form part of your body's primary defense against acid reflux.

Lastly, the pyloric sphincter is a ring of muscles that sits below your stomach. It opens to allow gastric emptying of your stomach's food contents into your small intestines, where further food processing can occur.

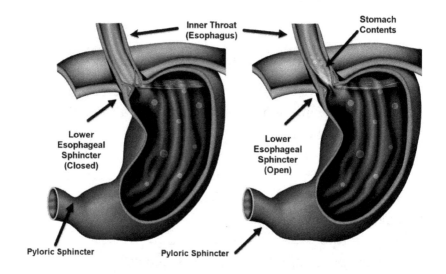

Figure 10

All three sphincters (lower esophageal, diaphragmatic, and pyloric) function automatically, based on biochemical signals sent from your stomach to the brain by way of the vagus nerve. This nerve is a pillar of your central nervous system and is your body's primary conduit for communications involving the brain and the gut. If instead, these muscles required conscious control, you would need to remember to tighten them every time you did a somersault, bent over, or hung upside down or you would get to see your lunch again when you forgot.

Relationship between Acidity and Your Sphincters

The lower esophageal and diaphragmatic sphincters are incredibly important as they contain the highly acidic hydrochloric acid that your stomach produces to efficiently break down your food into nutrients your body can absorb. Recall that typical measurements of acidity (pH scale) go from 1-14, with the smaller number being more powerful. The natural acidity of digestive juices in the human body is in the 1-3 range, which is slightly less acidic than battery acid.

The stomach can handle this highly corrosive fluid, as it is designed with thick inner lining and a protective mucosal layer. Other parts of your body, as you have observed, don't fare quite as well. As such, when this primary anti-reflux barrier fails you can experience inflammation or damage to the soft tissues of your nose, mouth, and throat.

The pyloric sphincter is equally important as after food is digested, it opens to permit transit of food contents into the small intestines. If this does not occur, or does not occur in a timely fashion, food contents remain in the stomach longer than necessary, leading to fermentation, gas, upset stomach, and indigestion.

As I stated, the muscles in these three sphincters are not under voluntary control and they function as an autonomic nervous system response. They are designed to close and prevent incidental exposure of stomach contents to the soft tissues outside of your stomach and to manage efficient flow of food contents through your digestive tract. Much as your eyelids automatically close when a particle is flying towards them, these sphincters close when abdominal acidity and pressure build up. This occurs naturally and automatically when your body is preparing to digest a meal.

Consequently, if your stomach acidity gets too low, your stomach will fail to signal your brain to open and close the sphincters at the right times and with sufficient pressure. As a result, the extended digestive process coupled with open sphincters will, as you might expect, lead to more reflux events. Of course, the frequency and severity of this exposure will dictate the symptoms and severity of the disease. Let's turn our attention to factors that can negatively impact the frequency and severity of this disease.

Causes of Low Acidity

Low stomach acid is actually a medical condition known as hypochlorhydria. As covered in the risk factors section, there are a number of potential precursors to acid reflux disease. Several of these risk factors can lead to low stomach acid, namely *(Leonard, "What is hypochlorhydria")*:

- **Diet** – A highly processed diet, or one that is high fat / sugar, or low food diversity can lead to an imbalance in the beneficial bacteria that aid in digestion and that make up your gut microbiome. Furthermore, as microbes in your digestive tract are essential to converting foods into essential minerals and vitamins, this can lead to vitamin and mineral deficiencies. Poor zinc absorption, in particular, is problematic as it is necessary for stomach acid production.
- **Chronic stress** – Studies have shown that when the body is under a state of persistent stress or depression the percentage of beneficial bacteria in your digestive tract declines and harmful pathogens quickly multiply to take their place *(Madison, "Stress, depression, diet")*.

- **Surgery** – Surgical procedures and associated medications can stress the body and can lead to reduced stomach acid. Gastric bypass surgeries additionally reduce the surface area of the stomach, thereby reducing the amount of stomach acid secreted.
- **Thyroid** – Thyroid dysfunction can lead to insufficient gastrin, the hormone that stimulates hydrochloric acid secretion.
- **Medications** – Antibiotics can similarly disrupt the bacteria balance in your gut.

If you are familiar with hypochlorhydria you may know that age is commonly cited as a risk factor. However, this is debatable as recent studies have demonstrated it is not age, but other lifestyle, medical, and disease factors that are more strongly correlated as being causal *(Goldshmiedt, "Effect of Age on Gastric Acid Secretion")*. No doubt, there are many more factors that can lead to low stomach acid. In truth, I would argue there is one risk factor that is by far the most impactful to acid reflux sufferers.

Acid Reflux Medications Are Making Your Reflux Worse

If you have been tracking up to this point, you know that low acidity results in low LES pressure. In fact, the lower the LES pressure, the more it allows for stomach contents to reflux out at greater intensity and frequency. Now, let's couple this with what we learned in the earlier chapters about acid reflux medications including antacids, H2 blockers, and PPIs. These medicines are designed to block the production of acids and lower your acidity to manage reflux symptoms...

I hope by now that you are going through the same shock that I went through when I came to this startling realization.

The very prescriptions that we are taking to help with reflux are progressively making it worse! Not only that, they are creating a co-dependency and ultimately escalating symptoms to a point where they can no longer be managed by the medications!

The below diagram illustrates this reflux cycle, which often begins with a little indigestion. After taking some antacids for relief, symptoms escalate to the point where many will visit a doctor. Upon confirming acid reflux symptoms, doctors often prescribe H2 blockers or PPIs.

Naturally, this escalates symptoms as the acid blocking medications compromise digestion and impair LES function. Over subsequent visits prescriptions are increased, LES function degrades further, and symptoms worsen. Additionally, as stomach acid is continually suppressed, it damages the balance of microbes in your gut, and further reduces digestive efficiency. Patients, unfortunately, spin around this loop until they find that the medications will no longer mitigate the symptoms.

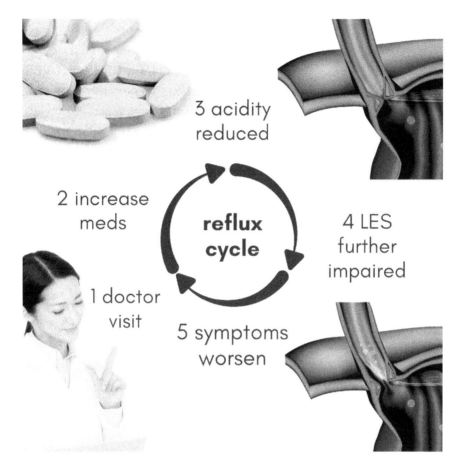

3 acidity
reduced

2 increase
meds

**reflux
cycle**

4 LES
further
impaired

1 doctor
visit

5 symptoms
worsen

Figure 11

We are unwittingly trading short term relief for long term system escalation and co-dependence on these medications. Now, understanding this cycle, I am convinced that my reflux disease and associated symptoms did not worsen on its own. Instead, it worsened due to my poor dietary choices and increasing levels of medications. This is a pattern that has been described by the thousands of individuals who visit my site monthly. Very few of which, I'm sure, would suspect that the very medicines prescribed by doctors to help with reflux, not only do not cure it, but make it significantly worse in the long term.

"ULTIMATELY, WHAT BEGAN AS A LITTLE INDIGESTION
AND IRRITATION, ENDED IN A FULL ONSLAUGHT OF MY
SENSES, MY SELF-WORTH, AND MY OUTLOOK ON LIFE. OVER
A 15 YEAR PERIOD, I WENT THROUGH THE PHASES OF OC-
CASIONAL INDIGESTION, TO ACID REFLUX, TO GERD, AND
THEN FULL ON SILENT REFLUX."

Now knowing what I know, I firmly believe that a slight change in diet would have eliminated the minor indigestion that caused me to reach for antacids and Pepto Bismol so many years ago. Had I merely understood how my body works, my symptoms would never have escalated to the point where I felt the need to visit the doctor. I would never have been prescribed the medications that escalated my symptoms so rapidly.

Salivary and esophageal bicarbonate response

Before we leave this topic of anti-reflux mechanisms, we have two more minor defenses to cover. Amazingly, your body is equipped with a fourth and fifth line of defense that can help to put out fires when your sphincters are asleep at the wheel.

As we covered in the demographics section, millions of people experience at least occasional reflux. Provided they have not progressed too far along the reflux cycle, these occasional bouts of heartburn are flushed by the body's fourth and fifth lines of defense.

Astonishingly, your body actually produces the equivalent of low dose antacids (bicarbonates) in your saliva and in your esophagus *(Helm, "Acid Neutralizing Capacity of Human Saliva")*. Both are triggered when the body detects acidity in the soft tissues of the throat or mouth. These salivary antacids are always present, however they increase thirty-two fold when the body detects errant acidity *(Tobey, "What Regulates Bicarbonate Secretion").* Your body's goal is to clear the acid and improve the damage resistance of the soft tissues.

Nonetheless, while these along with the mucosal response are effective in protecting soft tissues, they are no match for the more advanced forms of acid reflux that can be brought on by extended use of reflux medications or significant imbalance of digestive efficiency.

Digestion and the Microbiome

The digestive process involves a mind bogglingly complex symphony of biology and chemistry. In fact, the human body is often referred to as a microbiome, which describes the up to 5 pounds of microbes and viruses that live inside the body at any given time *(Univ. of Washington, "The Human Microbiome").*

If that surprises you, you will be shocked to learn that there are upwards of 100 trillion bacteria, over 1000 species and 7-9000 strains of those species in your body *(Varshauksi, "Probiotics Benefits + Myths").* Furthermore, the number of cells in your microbiome outnumbers your human cells by a factor of 10-1 *(Carpenter, "That Gut Feeling").* By cell count, we are indeed more bacteria than we are human!

What's more, the many organisms that live in the digestive tract have a mutualistic symbiotic relationship with us through our gut. Dr. Carpenter, in her article "That Gut Feeling" said "The human gut is an amazing piece of work. Often referred to as the "second brain," it is the only organ to boast its own independent nervous system, an intricate network of 100 million neurons embedded in the gut wall."

More broadly, the brain, gut, and microbiome form a highly collaborative and interconnected unit that govern your physical and mental state. As the gut-brain axis, a burgeoning field of medical research, has grown some have begun to refer to this triumvirate as "The Whole Brain!"

Benefits of the Microbiome

We commonly think of microorganisms as harmful, but in fact much of what lives in a healthy digestive tract is essential for life. Normally, there are a plethora of beneficial bacteria (probiotics) that help your body break down larger molecules like fats, proteins, and carbs into smaller molecules that are easier to absorb across the digestive tract.

I have shared that the psychological and social impacts of acid reflux were the most challenging for me. As I began to study this disease and its effects, it was clear to me that the b12, magnesium, and calcium deficiencies that I described had a profound effect on my mental and physical state. However, as I studied further I realized this only scratched the surface.

To my astonishment, I have since discovered that the bacteria in your microbiome work with your body to extract essential nutrients and to produce compounds and hormones such as serotonin, melatonin, dopamine, etc. These are the hormones that regulate your mood, sleep, and internal drive (Erika Ebbel. "Your Gut Microbiome"). The list of compounds that your body depends on your microbiome to produce is extensive and well beyond the scope of this book. Needless to say, these few examples alone highlight the importance of a balanced microbiome and how essential it is to your physical and mental wellbeing.

Additionally, up to 80% of your immune system is found in your gut. This is because the biggest potential threat to your body are things that you eat. In fact, everything you swallow is analyzed by your immune cells to determine if they are a threat. Under normal circumstances harmful pathogens are either destroyed by your stomach's high acidity or by your immune system. Quite interestingly, a well-balanced microbiome actually improves immune function and bolsters the lining of the stomach.

Damaging Your Microbiome

When your microbiome is compromised, however, it is unable to help your body digest foods. As a result, some food items, most commonly dairy, are identified by your digestive system as a threat. This triggers inflammation, which is a primary means for your body to isolate and attack invasive agents. The healing effects of inflammation are fine in short bursts. However, a persistent state of inflammation can erode the stomach wall and lead to a condition known as leaky gut. In this condition, harmful bacteria and food particles are able to bypass your immune system and the mucosal layer of your gut to enter your bloodstream.

As a result, swelling spreads to other areas of your body, setting off a chain reaction of issues. When inflammation reaches your brain you suffer cognitive issues (brain fog, memory problems, depression, anxiety, etc.), which add to your stress, and ultimately drives further imbalance to your microbiome. This is one of many self-destructive micro-cycles that make the broader reflux cycle so challenging.

Due to the gut-brain-microbiome connection, these micro-cycles are bi-directional. For instance, a poor diet can starve melatonin producing bacteria, which then affects your sleep. Also, poor sleep can disrupt the circadian rhythm of your microbiome. When you don't sleep, neither does your microbiome, leading to poor microbial health. Do this too often and you cause long term damage.

Lack of exercise can have a similar effect, in that it deprives your body of that peristalsis effect that can mobilize food through the gastrointestinal tract. This can be the difference between food stagnating and fermenting in your stomach vs the intestines or colon where fermentation should occur.

Your microbiome is constantly in flux, as it is dependent on the foods that you consume. If you don't eat enough fiber (vegetables, fruits, legumes, and whole grains) the beneficial bacteria in your gut that thrive on the otherwise indigestible fiber will die off, making room for other potentially less beneficial bacteria.

Similarly, if you eat the same types of foods day in, and day out the bacteria that specialize in helping you digest those foods will thrive, while others perish. In fact, you may have experienced over eating a food over a period and either becoming allergic, intolerant, or unable to eat it without discomfort. One cause is the proliferation of certain bacteria. If and when they get too numerous and are subsequently underfed, they can begin to attack the body. In response, the immune system can tag them and the associated food as hostile. The next time you eat the food, inflammation sets in and triggers reflux symptoms.

Lastly, certain medications, such as non-discriminate antibiotics can cause broad damage to the microbiome as they indiscriminately kill beneficial and non-beneficial bacteria. Far worse is the combination of antibiotics and acid suppressing medications as this significantly increases the risk of developing Small Intestinal Bacterial Overgrowth *(Revaiah, "Risk of SIBO in Patients Receiving PPI")*. As covered before, these microbial imbalances can result in damage to the stomach lining.

Hiatal Hernia

Lastly, I want to discuss the hiatal hernia. The hiatal hernia is a protrusion of the stomach into the esophagus. In my experience this is commonly diagnosed by those in the medical profession as a root cause. This is because a hiatal hernia is known to reduce LES pressure.

As I shared in my opening, I trusted my doctor's diagnosis of my hiatal hernia as the root cause of my reflux. As such, I didn't carry any hope of life without the disease. What I have since learned is, while a hiatal hernia does reduce the closing pressure of the LES, it does not necessarily render it inoperable. The Voice Institute of New York indicates a hiatal hernia decreases LES pressure by up to a one-third ("Silent Laryngopharyngeal Reflux").

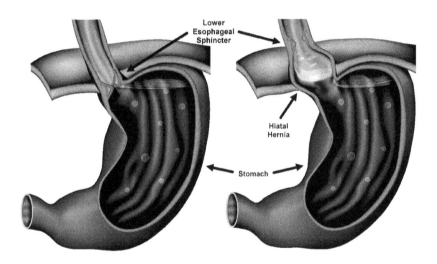

Figure 12

Unfortunately, as the medical profession often considers these hernias as a definitive root cause, there isn't much research that correlates the size of hernias with the reduction in pressure. Consequently, there aren't any clear diagnostics available that would help to determine if a hernia is too large to allow the LES to effectively close tight enough to prevent the occurrence of reflux. I don't take exception to the assertion that a hiatal hernia CAN be the root cause of reflux. I do, however, take exception to the idea that, when present, it IS the root cause. The key point that I want to make is, if you have a hiatal hernia, you do not need to give up hope as I did.

Summary

In this chapter we discussed the importance of acidity to proper anti-reflux barrier function and digestion. We explored the relationship of acid suppressing medications to the increasing severity and frequency of reflux events. Furthermore, we covered the connection between the gut, brain, and microbiome and its effects on your physical and mental wellbeing.

Your stomach is designed as a highly acidic environment to not only digest food, but to help maintain balance of this delicate ecosystem. If your stomach acid is too low, or other persistent risk factors are present it allows harmful pathogens and bacteria to multiply and overrun your digestive process *(Berg. "What is Betaine")*. Now that we understand the true root causes of acid reflux, we can divert our attention to the methods that can be used to resolve them.

Chapter 6

Phase I: Revise

It became an ongoing point of humor in my household. "Dad doesn't remember." My kids often wanted to hear a story from my childhood, or my wife would want the details of the day's events or a conversation with a family member. My longer term memories were less of a problem, but I was lucky if I could recall the high points of recent events, much more the fine details.

* * *

The following three chapters focus on the three acid reflux recovery phases: Revise, Restore, and Renew. I express the duration of these phases in a range as they largely depend on personal factors such as your diet, the extent of your digestive dysfunction, and your stomach's acidity.

Note, the approaches listed in each recovery phase are not a menu of options that can be cherry-picked. Instead, they are intended as a holistic approach to addressing the underlying root causes of acid reflux. Also, the recovery process itself is a bit like dropping a pebble into a pond. There are some ups and downs in the initial waves, but over time the waves turn into ripples, and the ripples smooth into the calm surface of the pond. Understanding this, a successful transition means paying attention to your body so you can adapt and adjust as necessary. For these reasons, I explain the rationale behind every approach so you have the requisite understanding that will support adjustments along the way. You may want to re-read this section a few times early in the transition.

Furthermore, you should think of these chapters as a daily checklist of activities. If you would like a condensed, printable, checklist version you can download it for free on my site at TheAcidRefluxGuy.com/transition. Additionally, links to the specific products that I used can be found at TheAcidRefluxGuy.com/resources.

Phase I: Revise Goal: Create a stable digestive environment to enable a smooth transition off of the reflux medications.
Duration: 2 weeks
Steps:

☐ **Continue taking existing acid reflux medications in this phase (if you are currently taking them)** - As you may have experienced in the past, it is nearly impossible to stop taking your acid reflux medication once you have entered the reflux cycle. To do this successfully and without discomfort you need three things: 1) closure of the esophageal sphincter 2) efficient digestion 3) minimal to no reflux events. Given this goal, you will want to spend the first two weeks of your recovery creating a baseline and significantly reducing the likelihood of reflux events. During this time, you will want to keep using medications, as you have been, so you do not experience reflux symptoms before you have a means to eliminate them. Also, you do not want to change too many things at once so you can tell what is going on in your body.

☐ **Eat plain foods and temporarily eliminate common reflux triggers from your diet (fatty foods, fried foods, processed foods, alcohol, high sugar, garlic, raw onions, spicy food, chocolate, citrus, caffeine, mint, tomato)** - This is simultaneously the hardest and MOST IMPORTANT step that you will take to support your transition. In this step, you need to temporarily eliminate all triggers from your diet. This will require that you get very picky about the things that you put in your body over the next few weeks. DO NOT skip this step. It is important to ensure you do everything you can to eliminate the potential for reflux events while you transition off of the medications. This dietary step will help to remove the effects of unknown (seemingly minor) inflammatory or allergy inducing food items and give you clarity and confidence that the transition is indeed successful. Without it, if you experience reflux symptoms due to trigger foods you will be uncomfortable and you will not be able to isolate the source of your discomfort. Furthermore, you will lack the confidence to complete the remaining steps to your recovery. If you need more time then add another week. It is more important to establish a solid baseline than it is to meet a time table.

Note this step recommends changes to your diet. For the most part, however, you should be able to eat your normal meals, so long as you leave out certain trigger items.

☐ **Take note of what you eat / drink and how it makes you feel; take note of and eliminate any additional food triggers that you identify** - The above step proactively eliminates acid reflux triggers that are fairly common. However, there may also be triggers that are unique to you. For me, it was dairy and bread. I actually didn't realize that bread triggered me until I spent some time baselining my diet. It just mixed in with the miscellaneous sea of reflux events. Now that I am back on track, I can eat both again with no issues.

☐ **Chew your food excessively, and do not overeat** - Experts say chew your food 32 times (or to a liquid). Even better if you can do that, but at a minimum strive to chew until you pulverize your food and then swallow. This will do two things for you 1) maximize coverage and time for enzymes in your saliva to start the pre-digestion process and 2) give your ailing digestive system a hand by breaking food down into more easily digested quantities.

☐ **Ensure you eat 2-3 hours before going to bed** - This allows time for your body to digest your dinner. Doing this, before laying horizontal, will reduce the likelihood and severity of nocturnal reflux events during your transition.

☐ **Add 'naturally fermented' foods to your daily diet (yogurt, pickles, sourdough, kimchi). For an internationally friendly list go to TheAcidRefluxGuy.com/fermented** - By the end of the restore phase your body needs to be able to efficiently digest food which will require help from the probiotics found in a healthy gut flora. A great source for this are fermented foods, because the fermentation process encourages growth of these helpful probiotic agents.

Note, while I do not have personal experience with Kombucha, it is widely reported as a very potent source of probiotics as well as for its effectiveness in killing harmful bacteria. This may be especially helpful if you have SIBO.

Note, if you do not eat fermented foods regularly, you should slowly introduce them to your diet. Use a wide variety of these important probiotic sources to increase the diversity of your gut flora. Ideally you can work up to eating them daily during your transition.

Note, some foods such as pickles often use modern fermentation processes which strip the product of its probiotic qualities. To guard against this, look for the phrase 'naturally fermented.'

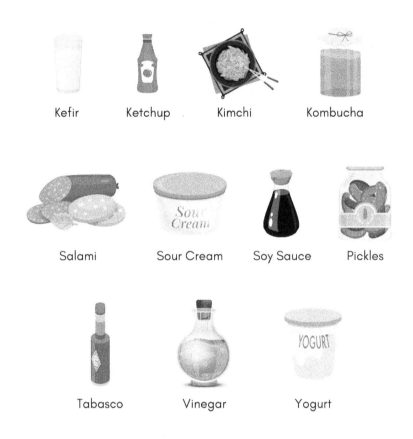

Kefir   Ketchup   Kimchi   Kombucha

Salami   Sour Cream   Soy Sauce   Pickles

Tabasco   Vinegar   Yogurt

Figure 13

☐ **Add 35-50 grams of natural dietary fiber sources to your daily diet including fruits, vegetables, and legumes)** - Prebiotics are important sources of nutrients for the probiotics that we are introducing in this phase. Support optimal balance by introducing fiber rich foods daily including fruits, vegetables, legumes, and whole grains. If you do not have these in your diet, the newly introduced probiotics will starve and die off, thus limiting your recovery. Adding these items consistently to your diet will encourage regrowth of beneficial bacteria and help to restore your physical and mental wellbeing.

Note, aim to eat enough fruits, vegetables, and legumes daily to obtain 35-50 grams of fiber. This is different than eating 35-50 grams of fruits, vegetables, and legumes daily.

Note, during your transition avoid high concentrations of processed sugars and pre-packaged foods as they serve as a prebiotic food source for harmful bacteria.

☐ **Eat yogurt after meals (if you have become lactose intolerant over time, try and re-introduce later after your digestion improves)** - During my transition, I ate yogurt for breakfast and a half cup of yogurt after meals. It provides a soothing / calming effect on digestion. Also, I should note that, like me, you may have developed a lactose intolerance over the years. It turns out that restoring your digestive balance may restore your ability to enjoy milk based products. So if you try yogurt and find that you cannot tolerate it, give it a few weeks and try again. If you are like me, you will find that you can resume enjoying treats such as parfaits. Here are a couple treats that I still enjoy:

Yogurt with Sliced Apples & Granola

- For breakfast, 1 ½ cups of plain non-fat yogurt (or just half a cup after meals)
- Add unsweetened apple sauce to taste
- Finely slice apples to add texture, flavor, and to serve as a filler
- For breakfast add some old fashioned oats so the meal will be filling
- Top with granola to taste. Note, if you plan to eat this often it is best to avoid adding a lot of granola as it can be

a high sugar source which feeds less desirable bacteria in your gut

Yogurt with Frozen Blueberries & Almonds

- For breakfast, 1 ½ cups of plain non-fat yogurt (or just half a cup after meals)
- For breakfast add old fashioned oats so the meal will be filling
- Pour in frozen blueberries for interesting contrast, cold therapy, and taste!
- Add some plain unsalted almonds for texture and protein
- Top with granola to taste

Sliced apples with Almonds and Raisins

- For breakfast, dice one red apple into small bites
- Add three teaspoons of plain non-fat yogurt and mix to cover the apples evenly
- Add raisins, almonds and a little cinnamon to taste. Note, cinnamon is a great prebiotic and unfortunately a common reflux trigger so you might avoid this early in your transition

☐ **Take Vitamin B12 and Magnesium supplements daily (if needed)** – Long term use of these drugs are known to lead to several deficiencies including magnesium, calcium, and vitamin B12. Vitamin B12 and magnesium supplements are readily available over the counter. I took 3000mcg B12 gummies and 100 mg Magnesium Citrate. You can take the B12 and Magnesium supplements daily to restore these extremely vital vitamins. In my personal experience the positive effects on my sense of touch, vision, and mood were immediate and signifi-cant!

Note, I don't recommend taking Calcium supplements as they are an alkaline and counteract new acid production *(Berg. "What is Betaine")*. Given this, it is best to restore your digestive efficiency using the techniques discussed in this book, which will in turn allow your body to properly process calcium again.

☐ **Get a thermal cup and drink lots of warm water throughout the day** - Drinking lots of warm liquids between meals promotes digestion and can help to break up accumula-tion of stomach contents or mucus in the throat.

Note, I emphasize *between* meals as drinking large quanti-ties during meals can dilute digestive efficiency.

☐ **Near the end of week 2, optionally take an essential enzyme capsule with meals** - If you have successfully re-base-lined your diet and removed triggers, over two weeks' time, then you can optionally introduce digestive enzymes with meals. To do so, take one 500 mg capsule in the middle of meals. The purpose is to get a sense for its effects on your di-gestion process. If you are like most, you will feel a definitive improvement in your symptoms. It's important to wait until you are confident in your ability to isolate triggering events before introducing this supplement. This will help you to bet-ter isolate the effects of adding digestive enzymes and further build confidence in a successful transition.

Chapter 7

Phase II: Restore

I often skipped lunch before important meetings and presentations. If I didn't, invariably my voice would fail on me, zapping my confidence for the talk. Rather than concentrate on my key messages, I worried that people would observe the change in my voice quality and interpret it as nerves or lack of confidence.

* * *

Phase II: Restore Goal: Leverage supplements to temporarily simulate the body's normal digestive function, restore sphincter function, eliminate indigestion, rebalance gut flora, and enable you to stop taking your reflux medications.

Duration: 4-6 weeks

Steps:

□ **Take one 500 mg apple cider vinegar capsule with meals** - Apple Cider Vinegar supplements are rich in enzymes and prebiotics that promote rapid return of beneficial bacteria in your stomach *(McDermott, "Can you use ACV to treat Acid*

Reflux"). They also contain acetic acid, which additionally can help kill pathogens, including bad bacteria that multiply in low acid conditions.

Note, if you struggle to take pills then consider extending Phase I and allow the reduced triggers, high fiber (prebiotic) and fermented foods (probiotics) to take effect. This will hopefully have a positive effect on inflammation in your throat.

Note, I recommend taking this supplement in the middle of your meal as it is best when there is something in your stomach.

Note, I DO NOT recommend taking Apple Cider Vinegar in liquid form, even diluted or consumed using a straw. As it is acidic, it can corrode tooth enamel and the soft tissues of your throat when taken orally *(Leonard, "Does ACV Help with Acid Reflux").*

☐ **Take one 500 mg essential enzyme capsule with meals** - This supplement helps to compensate for low acidity and poor digestion by helping the body break down proteins, fats, milk sugars, fiber and carbohydrates. This vegetable based supplement also reports the benefit of relieving lactose intolerance through the introduction of beneficial enzymes. This certainly matches my experience.

Note, I recommend taking this supplement in the middle of your meal as it is best when there is something in your stomach.

☐ **Take one or more 650 mg betaine hydrochloride + pepsin capsules with meals, according to size and complexity of the meal. Increase with subsequent meals until it controls your symptoms. If you notice discomfort, take less for a similar meal next time** – Betaine is a nutritional compound extracted from food sources like grains or beets. Betaine HCl is an acidic version of betaine that works in the same way as hydrochloric acid (HCl) in your stomach *(Dr Ruscio, "Betaine HCl")*. Quite often, insufficient acid production is paired with insufficient pepsin production so be sure your variety of betaine HCl contains pepsins as these help to break down protein.

This supplement supports digestion, helps to support healthy gut function, and safely restore normal gastric acidity *(Carolina Total Wellness, "How to Support Optimal Stomach Acid for Good Digestion")*. More importantly, this along with increased intra-abdominal pressure, are the triggers your body needs to signal your sphincters to close *(Berg. "What is Betaine")*. Additionally, acidity is required to signal the pyloric sphincter to efficiently and effectively release stomach contents into the small intestines. Lastly, achieving optimal stomach acidity helps your body to rebalance your microbiome as beneficial microbes thrive in the naturally high acidity found in the gut; non-beneficial microbes are allowed to flourish in the presence of insufficient acidity. These factors are key to enable you to stop taking your prescription or over-the-counter reflux medications and antacids.

That said, not everyone will need to take HCl as a part of their recovery. Consider this section as a guide to test if it will be beneficial for you. There isn't a standard recommended dose of Betaine so plan to start with one 650 mg hydrochloride capsule in the middle of your largest meal for the day (usually dinner). I emphasize taking this supplement in the middle of your meal as it is best when there is something in your stomach. Take this first dose with a meal containing protein. If you do not feel an improvement in your digestion, try two capsules the next day, with a similar sized meal. Because the ideal dose depends on personal factors such as your acidity and meal complexity this will require some experimentation and some patience. That said, you will know if you are taking enough if it is helping to control your reflux symptoms.

The dose for each meal will also vary according to the size and complexity of the meal. For example, I often took 2-3 with dinner, 4-5 for very high protein meals, and 1-2 for breakfast and lunch. Over time, by paying attention to your body, you will gain a sense for the right dose. The supplements are not required for light snacks.

In his book "Why Stomach Acid Is Good for You" Dr. Wright indicates "the most effective dose of betaine HCl is 5 to 7 of the 650 mg capsules per meal, with pepsin *(Wright, "Why Stomach Acid Is Good for You)."* Increase by one pill each day until you reach 5-7, feel a warming sensation in your gut, or have a heartburn sensation, whichever comes first. The heartburn or warming sensations are your signal to decrease by one pill for similar sized meals, as your body has sufficient acidity. When you find the ideal dose, continue taking the supplements with up to three meals daily. Remember, there is no need to further increase your dose provided the supplements are helping to manage your symptoms.

In the coming days and weeks, as your body naturally increases stomach acid production, the aforementioned sensations will be the signal to further wean off of the hydrochloride by one capsule. Note that some individuals never feel the warmth sensation. If this is you, then your test is whether or not the supplements are helping to improve your digestion. If not, then you may need to increase by one capsule. Additionally, every few days try decreasing by one capsule per meal if digestive issues return, then add them back. The goal is continue reducing the dose until you reach zero capsules with meals. This will be your trigger to move on to Phase III.

Note, those with ulcers or inflammatory conditions should NOT use HCl. Individuals taking medicines such as steroids or anti-inflammatories (Aspirin, Motrin, Advil, etc..) should not use HCl as the combination can damage the gastrointestinal lining.

Note, by my second week on the supplements, I found that I experienced a lot of gas and the urge to belch a lot after meals. However, by the third week it subsided.

Note, if a single capsule of HCl gives you heartburn then you may have sufficient stomach acidity. However, if a single capsule of HCl gives you the warmth sensation, it is possible that you are still deficient in stomach acid. Paradoxically, Dr. Wright points out that "adverse symptoms are most likely to occur in individuals with the lowest levels of stomach acid. This is because these people are the most likely to have atrophic gastritis (a thinned out stomach lining). When HCl supplementation is not feasible, gradually increasing quantities of lemon juice (citric acid) or vinegar (acetic acid) will often relieve some or even all of the symptoms *(Wright, "Why Stomach Acid Is Good for You)."* If you find similar results with these methods, then your acidity may indeed be sufficient. If this is the case, then your focus should be on the recommended improvements to your digestive balance including the introduction of probiotics / prebiotic foods, and use of digestive enzymes.

☐ **During the transition, if you notice a return of reflux symptoms or stomach discomfort, this is a signal to reduce the number of HCl capsules you take with meals by one; when you reach zero move to Renew phase** - You may reach a point where you do not need to take as many HCl capsules, as doing so creates excess acid, which results in a bit of your typical reflux symptoms. If this occurs, simply reduce your dose of HCl with meals going forward. This is a sign that your natural acidity is returning and that soon you will be able to get off of the supplements.

☐ **Stop taking acid reflux medications (h2 blockers, PPIs, and antacids)** - The supplements we have added will temporarily simulate your body's normal digestive function by balancing acidity and supplying needed digestive enzymes. This should restore your sphincter function, address indigestion, and enable you to stop taking your reflux medications effective immediately. If you are not there yet, you may need to increase the dose of the hydrochloride supplement.

Note, you should always consult a doctor before stopping, starting, or altering the dose of any prescription medication.

☐ **Continue taking the Vitamin B12 and Magnesium supplements daily (if needed)** - Continue taking these through the remainder of phase 2.

☐ **Continue eating your plain, trigger free diet** - Continue your trigger free meals through the remainder of phase 2.

☐ **Continue taking notes and making adjustments based on reflux symptoms that you observe** - Continue noting any symptoms and adjust as necessary. Symptoms continue to reduce as your digestive health improves.

☐ **Continue eating the high fiber prebiotic foods** – Continue eating the high fiber prebiotic foods as this will encourage regrowth of beneficial bacteria and help to restore your physical and mental wellbeing.

☐ **Continue eating the fermented foods** - Continue eating fermented foods as this meal diversity will help build a foundation for solid digestion and will encourage regrowth of beneficial bacteria and help to restore your physical and mental wellbeing.

☐ **Continue eating yogurt after meals** - Continue eating yogurt to stabilize symptoms and introduce beneficial probiotics and encourage regrowth of beneficial bacteria and help to restore your physical and mental wellbeing.

Chapter 8

Phase III: Renew

My boss and I met to share some initiative plans with a Vice President of one of my company's business segments. It was a very cordial and positive meeting. I can't remember what specifically was said, but I do remember that, at some point, I broke out into spontaneous sweats. My face was pouring as though my sports headband had reached saturation and was now sponging down my face. I did a quick scan of the room to see if any napkins or paper towels were left in the meeting from a lunch meeting. No luck. Despite the fact that I was the only presenter, I abruptly got up and walked to the bathroom where I spent a few minutes trying to regain my composure. When I returned, I resumed the meeting as if nothing had happened. They were kind enough not to comment on my shame.

* * *

P hase III: Renew Goal: Stop taking the supplements and slowly reintroduce your normal diet.
Duration: 2+ weeks
Steps:

☐ Once you have reached zero HCl capsules in the restore phase, you can stop taking all supplements – This is the trigger to end Phase II. Contrary to your current lifetime subscription of acid reflux medications, you do not need to take the supplements for life. They serve the short term purpose of facilitating a quick and smooth transition off of reflux medications while allowing your body to rebuild digestive health. When you have reduced your HCl down to zero, then you can discontinue all of the supplements.

☐ Slowly, reintroduce foods that you have not eaten during the transition phase. You may notice that foods that you could not digest in the past no longer present an issue - I recommend that you take it easy here. As you reintroduce foods, take note how they affect you. I found that dairy and bread were back on the menu. Your experience may vary. If some foods still give you trouble, look into a probiotic that targets that specific intolerance. Probiotics with a minimum 50 Billion Colony Forming Units (CFU) and that are Enteric Coated, are best as this will delay release until the supplement reaches the small intestine *(Dr. Mike, "Probiotics Benefits + Myths")*.

☐ Hold onto the supplements in case you start to feel some of the early symptoms of reflux again in the future. If you catch it early, a day or two on the supplements and some yogurt can put you back in balance - As noted above, you are not immune to acid reflux now that you have recovered. As such, you do need to take care to avoid the risk factors that you got you in this situation in the first place. If it happens again, the difference is that you are now armed with the information you need to quickly get back on track.

☐ Continue the high fiber diet (prebiotic) and fermented foods (probiotic) to maintain a robust microbiome balance — Now that you have recovered, it is important to ensure you stay that way. While ok to reduce the quantity, keeping these items in your diet on a regular basis is important to further build and maintain healthy digestive balance.

☐ Celebrate! But take care to avoid the risk factors that initiated your reflux in the first place. For a refresher, you can review the epidemiology chapter / risk factors chapter - Congrats! You are now back your normal self before ever having entered this crazy reflux cycle.

☐ Acid reflux disease affects more than one in eight people globally, so chances are you will know someone that you can share this information with. Remember, sharing is caring! - Who do you know that is struggling with acid reflux? If this approach has helped you, be sure and tell them what you've done. Drop me a line as well! I would love to hear from you. I'm on a mission to positively impact 100,000 people and you play an important role in reaching that goal!

Chapter 9

Ninja Tips & Tricks

My wife suffered my random muscle spasms in bed for almost 15 years! I was later vindicated when I found that this was a common side effect of low magnesium and calcium (carpopedal spasms). In fact, my wife's sleep has improved greatly since healing my reflux. No more inadvertent kicks, no more gurgling, coughing hacking fits, and no more disrupted breathing!

* * *

As you have learned in this book, the most effective method for dealing with the side effects of acid reflux is by addressing the root causes including low acidity and poor digestive efficiency. In the meantime, however, there are some things you can do to reduce your discomfort. The following techniques, when performed consistently and in combination can really help to take the edge off.

Before we cover the tips for managing mucus, battling breath issues, and solving sleep problems, I want to note there are several general tips that will have positive effects across each of the three issues. They are already covered in the Revise, Restore, and Renew section, so I will not cover them again here (i.e. eating yogurt, avoiding triggers, drinking warm water, and eating high fiber and fermented foods).

If you would like a condensed, printable, checklist version of the below tips you can download it for free on my site at TheAcidRefluxGuy.com/NinjaTips. Additionally, links to the specific products that I used can be found at TheAcidRefluxGuy.com/resources.

Managing Mucus

Easily one of the most infuriating symptoms of silent reflux is the seemingly endless stream of MUCUS! Oftentimes, it is accompanied by a slight burning sensation or a salty, sweet, sour, or vinegar taste and smell. Contrary to your stomach, which has a *persistent* barrier against high acidity and digestive enzymes, your nose and throat favor a *just-in-time* approach. When your body senses the presence of acids or acid vapors in these sensitive areas, it triggers the release of mucus.

Pepsins are the Culprit

The constant presence of mucus is intensely annoying, however you may not realize that it is not your primary irritant. The credit for much of the discomfort caused by the mucus actually belongs to an accumulation of pepsins. Pepsins are digestive enzymes that are responsible for breaking down proteins. During reflux events they can get trapped and accumulate in the soft tissues of your throat, nose, and mouth during reflux events.

Pepsins are great when helping to digest your food, however they are not so great when they are digesting you. Normally, they are activated by the acidity in your stomach. However, they can additionally be activated by acid vapors and even acidic foods and drinks.

At the worst stage of my reflux, I suffered from this seemingly endless onslaught of mucus. Worse, though, was the constant burning pins and needles sensation in the roof of my mouth and my lips. Over a couple of weeks, by faithfully adhering to the supplement schedule, the burning sensations disappeared entirely.

Now that you understand pepsins and how they accumulate over time, you can appreciate the importance of having a consistent routine that will rid these sensitive areas of your nose, throat, and mouth of these digestive enzymes.

There are several methods you can employ to reduce the presence of pepsins and proactively discourage their accumulation including:

☐ **Eat raw fruits and vegetables that are high in fiber** – This has a dual benefit of providing prebiotics that will nourish beneficial bacteria in your gut and help to neutralize odor producing bacteria in your mouth.

☐ **Chew your food excessively to improve pre-digestion** - Try excessively chewing your food, which allows your body to maximize pre-digestion. This will help your body to more efficiently break down foods as it flows through your digestive system.

☐ **Eat 2-3 hours before laying down for bed** – Make it a point to eat at least 2-3 hours before laying down so that your food is more fully digested. This will reduce the likelihood of nocturnal reflux events, which occur more frequently due to being in a horizontal position.

☐ **Sleep on your left side** – Numerous reflux studies cover the benefits of sleeping on your left side due to the body's asymmetrical anatomy. This position is shown to improve digestion and reduce the occurrence of reflux events. Personally, I found that rotating between laying on my side and my stomach was much preferred over sleeping on my back. Invariably, when I did sleep on my back I would wake up in the middle of a night choking on stomach contents.

☐ **Try elevating your body with a wedge pillow** - Under normal conditions, the body naturally produces about 1.5 quarts of mucus daily. Acid reflux can push this into overdrive. When we sleep, this can accumulate due to the fact that the body's saliva flow virtually ceases during sleep. Consequently, we swallow less. To combat this, try elevating your upper body with a wedge pillow.

☐ **Clear your nose and throat** - Given the presence of pepsins, it is important to clear your nose and throat regularly. Guys know how to do both instinctively as we have been 'hocking loogies' since the age of 4. The best times to do this proactive throat clearing is in the mornings when you wake up, potentially after meals, and before you go to bed.

☐ **Use a saline solution** - Reflux sufferers can deal with indigestion, which allows for stomach contents to reflux into the esophagus and trigger the mucus response. Nasal solutions are available over the counter and can be used to help clear mucus from your nose and nasal passage. Not all nasal sprays can be used on a regular basis, so be sure to follow the warning labels and instructions for best and safe results.

These methods will not eliminate your mucus, but they can help to manage the annoying by-products. Practice them on a consistent basis for best results.

Battling Breath Issues

Most people are confused as to the source of their breath issues. Intuitively, we think we must have some bad chemistry going on in our mouth. After all, it is seemingly the source of the offending odor. Additionally, the fact that you can't consistently or effectively smell your own breath leads you to wonder if it is bad or if it's in your head. Then there is a growing fear, if it is bad, how close do others have to be to smell it?

So let's just both agree that this topic is a bit gross. That gives us license to discuss this frankly... There are two reasons you can't consistently smell your own breath. The first is your brain is designed to ignore things that you are familiar with such as your own smell. This is one of the brain's adaptive mechanisms to help you avoid sensory overload. Second, breath is more easily detected by your nose when scented molecules break down in air.

So, the easiest way to determine if your breath has an odor is to lick the back of your hand. Let it dry and then give it a sniff. There are many different odors and interpretations of these odors. You can google until your heart's content. That said, if you do detect an odor it does not necessarily mean that others can smell it. The best way, while extremely embarrassing, is to ask someone or you can get a clinical diagnosis, called an organoleptic measurement.

Now, we can talk about methods to improve the freshness of your breath. Below are a couple of methods that I have found to be fairly effective.

☐ **Try neutralizing your mouth with a pinch of baking soda, antacids, or bicarbonate mouthwash (do not swallow)** – Through the course of the day, stomach contents can find their way into your throat and mouth where they will accumulate, unless you take action. Try a pinch or two of baking soda as a mouthwash. It will quickly dissolve in your mouth and you can gargle it and then spit as you would a traditional mouthwash. Alternatively, if you still have antacids around, you can use these as well. Lastly, you could try a bicarbonate mouthwash. Treat each of these as you would a typical mouthwash and do not swallow, as this would lower acidity and can contribute to the reflux cycle.

☐ **Use a baking soda as toothpaste** – Typically toothpastes use mint to give you that clean feeling, but can trigger a mucus response and relaxation of the LES. Alternatively, use a sparing amount of baking soda as a toothpaste. As a side benefit, I find that this leaves a better clean than most toothpastes. Much like you feel after a good scrubbing from the dentist!

☐ **Brush all the surfaces of your mouth with an electric toothbrush** - When brushing, it's important to realize that you should clear accumulated stomach contents from your mouth. To do this, use an electric toothbrush to brush all the surfaces of your mouth including your inner cheek, gums, your tongue, and the roof of your mouth.

☐ **Use a tongue scraper** - If you don't have a tongue scraper, get one! The vast majority of sulfur bacteria in your mouth actually live on your tongue. Brushing your tongue just moves them around. Scraping, in contrast, will dislodge those little buggers!

☐ **Brush teeth 30 minutes after eating** - It is ok to brush your teeth multiple times per day. Do this after neutralizing with baking soda or 30 minutes after eating or a reflux event to avoid brushing when your mouth is the most acidic.

☐ **Stimulate your salivary defenses with moisturizing gels and oral lozenges** - I will admit, I do not have personal experience with this particular method. That said, it lines up very well with my research and understanding of your body's natural reflux defense. As covered in this book, your body's salivary response creates bicarbonates which help in neutralizing acids. Moisturizing gels and oral lozenges have been shown to increase your saliva's acid neutralization capacity.

Solving Sleep Problems

☐ **If you are vitamin B12 deficient, try taking B12 supplements** – If, after reviewing the symptoms described in the Acid Reflux Disease chapter, you believe you have a B12 deficiency, this tip may help to restore your sleep. For years, I suffered with sleep deprivation. After sleeping for +8 hours, I would wake feeling groggy, with brain fog, headaches, and not feeling rested. I later discovered that two side effects of my acid reflux were causing my sleep issues. These were nocturnal reflux, leading to coughing fits, and vitamin B12 deficiencies. Vitamin B12 is essential to keeping your nerve cells healthy. Its absence can lead to neurological issues including poor sleep. Taking B12 supplements, as covered in the Revise chapter, may help you to sleep more restfully.

☐ **If you are magnesium deficient, try taking magnesium supplements** – Magnesium has been shown to aid with sleep by helping the body and brain reach a state of calm and relaxation. It also helps to manage melatonin levels which help to moderate sleep cycles *(Jennings, "How Magnesium Can Help You Sleep")*.

☐ **Try melatonin supplements** – Before resolving my reflux, I did find that the over the counter drug melatonin was fairly effective in helping with a restful night's sleep. This particular drug I find quite finicky, as some people do not notice its effects at all, while others are knocked out with a very low dose. For me, it took 30-40mg to take effect. While on melatonin, I woke each morning feeling significantly better than I had in years. In comparison to my sleep now, this is merely an 80% solution.

Note, melatonin is also reported to have a positive effect on lower esophageal sphincter function, which may have also contributed to my more restful sleep. I can't say that it noticeably reduced the occurrence of waking with a mouth full of mucus and stomach contents. Nonetheless, I found it an effective short term tool to improve my sleep. I still keep it above my bed, even now, for the rare occasion that I can't seem to sleep.

Summary

These are a few tips that you can use to manage breath, sleep, and mucus issues while you are working through your transition. Practice them consistently for best results as the effects of reflux that contribute to these issues are largely cumulative in nature. In the same way, practicing these techniques over time will lead to a cumulative improvement in the management of these symptoms.

Chapter 10

Conclusion

Despite an incomplete understanding of the situation, I felt a gravity set in. My wife felt it too and she consequently grilled the doctor, looking for an alternative to a lifelong prescription. She asked the Doctor "What are his choices?" To which, he replied "Well, your choices are continued throat irritation and the possibility of esophageal cancer... or the prescription. Surgical techniques have only shown to last a few years." Given those two options, the choice was clear. Having grown up in a medical household I trusted western medications and, while the doctor never said this, I thought the medications would heal me. Nonetheless, the drive back to our apartment was somber and contemplative. Somehow, I had a feeling that this was a defining moment in the course of my life.

* * *

In my dedication, I shared that "the sequence of events that led to my discovery of the methods, which led to my healing, and the authorship of this book could only have come from God." I say this as this book, website, recovery, and the research that underpinned it would never have happened were it not for one fateful moment.

Over the 2019 Christmas break, an out of state friend came to visit our family. At one point, she noticed I was massaging my fingers and asked "Why are you doing that?" To which I responded, "Sometimes my fingers tingle and this helps them feel better. Probably too much time on the computer." To my complete and utter astonishment, she replied, "Do you have acid reflux?" She then went on to explain this as a common side effect of long term acid reflux medications due to b12 deficiency. As you might imagine, this seemingly random, yet spot on observation peaked my interest. I spent the next day in intense research reading riveting articles like "Depression, Hematologic Parameters, and Blood Levels of Vitamin B12 in Patients With Laryngopharyngeal Reflux Under Use of Proton Pump Inhibitors." I sought to understand the tie to b12 deficiency. This ultimately led me to the root causes of the disease and its treatments. After which, I had the beginnings of a framework that I would follow to hopefully eliminate my reflux for good.

Now, as I write these words, I am a few days from January 16th, 2020 my Independence Day from acid reflux medications. It was the last day that I took acid reflux medications. It was also the day the supplements that I ordered arrived in the mail. I eagerly took them that evening with dinner. The next morning, I woke feeling better than I had in nearly 15 years. For once, my mouth and throat were clear and I felt like I had a full night's sleep.

As I was getting ready for work that morning, I came to a conclusion that I had to share this information with as many people as possible. I called in a day of vacation. I then purchased TheAcidRefluxGuy.com and feverishly tapped out the first blog post! You know, I still have the last bottles of prescription medications that I ever filled:

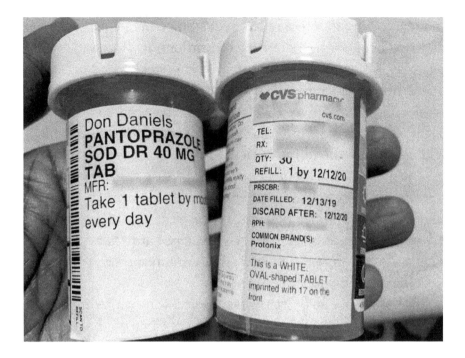

Figure 14

After reading this text, you should have a solid understanding of how these medications work and how they contribute to the reflux cycle. Ultimately, reflux is a digestive disorder that needs to be addressed by closing your sphincters, and rebuilding digestive efficiency. If you have experienced the long term side effects of this disease, you now know that vitamin supplements can help to quickly re-introduce these vital nutrients to your body.

Furthermore, it is my hope that, with a thorough understanding of this disease and its risk factors you can find healing and avoid relapsing by falling victim to the risk factors that started you down this path the first time. Since my recovery, I have reintroduced all the foods that I ate prior to starting my recovery.

That said, I do have a hiatal hernia, which makes me more sensitive to changes in my digestion. I also know from looking at my past experiences that a high sugar diet is a risk factor that can push me into a reflux cycle. Since my recovery, I have had two occasions where I have overdone it. One was on my birthday, where over the course of the weekend, I ate large quantities of pie, brownies, and candy. After several days trying to understand why I was experiencing a mucus response again, after being +6 months symptom free, it dawned on me. I had re-entered the reflux cycle.

The good news is that a couple of days on the supplements put me back on track. Another occasion was over the holiday break. As a Christmas present, I received a tub of sour strips, my absolute favorite candy. Let's just say, I ate a good amount. This time, when some of my symptoms returned, I knew to supplement for a couple of days.

All that being said, I later discovered that while my symptoms were gone, I still had not reached optimal gut balance. To resolve this, I ramped my fiber intake up to the 35-50 grams that I covered in the transition plan. That did the trick. I firmly believe that keeping prebiotic and probiotic sources in your daily diet is one of the most important steps to build resilience in your gut. Now, ff you find that you are unable to maintain balance then you might consider probiotic supplements, such as those at TheAcidRefluxGuy.com/Resources.

The relapses that I experienced are reminder that the very same risk factors that started my reflux so long ago could still start me down the path of the reflux cycle. To that end, I continue to enjoy all my favorite snacks and deserts on a regular basis but I do so in moderation and against the backdrop of a health promoting diet rich in pre and probiotics.

With exception of the brief setbacks I have mentioned, I lived the last year free of my reflux medications, supplements, and symptoms. I no longer have anxiety or break into the cold sweats that plagued the last 15 years of my existence. My voice, mind, and my vision are clear. I do not have to worry about falling asleep while driving due to extreme fatigue. No more waking up in the middle of the night in a coughing and gagging fit. I am finally free after 15 years of torment.

On a whim, I checked to see if I still had the text trail where I tried to cancel the automatic renewal of prescription medications with the pharmacy. Sadly, I couldn't cancel via text and had to call in. I have enclosed pictures of both as a fitting memorial to this chapter in my life. You can see the timestamp, about 2 weeks after starting the supplements. Just 6 weeks later I was completely off of the supplements as well. My reflux story began more than 15 years ago when I started taking medications. This past year, I turned the page on the last chapter of that book, and I sincerely hope that by using the methods in this book you can do the same.

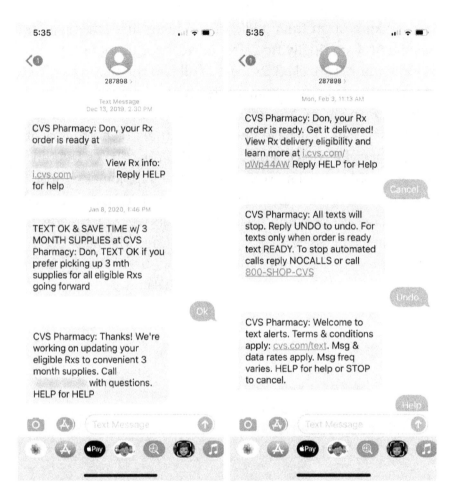

Figure 15

Lastly, I am on a mission to positively impact 100,000 people. If I have inspired, helped, informed or otherwise assisted you in anyway, let me know by giving me a follow on any of the below platforms. If I have yet to do so, then take advantage of the daily tips available on these sites!

Follow me at:

TheAcidRefluxGuy.com/Instagram
TheAcidRefluxGuy.com/Pinterest

TheAcidRefluxGuy.com/YouTube
TheAcidRefluxGuy.com/Twitter

OR

Join the TheAcidRefluxGuy.com/BookMailingList. This page has been set up for those that have purchased this book and it will get you exclusive, early, free, and discounted access to new content!

Chapter 11

Works Cited

Acid Reflux Disease

Dr S. J. O. Veldhuyzen van Zanten. "Validation of a 7–point Global Overall Symptom scale to measure the severity of dyspepsia symptoms in clinical trials." Wiley, onlinelibrary.wiley.com/doi/full/10.1111/j.1365-2036.2006.02774.x. Accessed 7, September 2020.

Matthew Solan. "Can a heartburn drug cause cognitive problems?" Harvard Health Publishing Harvard Medical School, https://www.health.harvard.edu/blog/can-heartburn-medication-cause-cognitive-problems-201603219369. Accessed 10, January 2021.

Thawin Srinutta et. al. "Proton pump inhibitors and hypomagnesemia: A meta-analysis of observational studies." National Library of Medicine National Center for Biotechnology Information, https://pubmed.ncbi.nlm.nih.gov/31689852/. Accessed 10, January 2021.

Yousef Nassar et. al. "Proton-pump Inhibitor Use and Fracture Risk: An Updated Systematic Review and Meta-analysis." US National Library of Medicine National Institutes of Health, https://www.ncbi.nlm.nih.gov/pmc/articles/PMC6135649/. Accessed 10, January 2021.

Epidemiology

Andrea Maria Campagnolo. "Laryngopharyngeal Reflux: Diagnosis, Treatment, and Latest Research." SciElo, https://www.scielo.br/scielo.php?script=sci_art-text&pid=S1809-48642014000200184. Accessed 13, December 2020.

Annelise Madison. "Stress, depression, diet, and the gut microbiota: human–bacteria interactions at the core of psychoneuroimmunology and nutrition." US National Library of Medicine, https://www.ncbi.nlm.nih.gov/pmc/articles/PMC7213601/. Accessed 4, Feb 2021

Chutkan, Robynne. "The Microbiome Solution." Tantor Media, Inc. May 16, 2016

Dr. Guarner. "MAP OF DIGESTIVE DISORDERS & DISEASES." World Gastroenterology Organisation, https://www.worldgastroenterology.org/UserFiles/file/wdhd-2008-map-of-digestive-disorders.pdf. Accessed 13, December 2020.

Dr. Ramalinga Kedika. "Hiatal Hernia – A Very Common Condition." Medical Center Health System, https://mchodessa.com/fitness/hiatal-hernia-a-very-common-condition/. Accessed 5, January 2021.

Jérôme R. Lechien et al. "Impact of laryngopharyngeal reflux on subjective and objective voice assessments: a prospective study ", https://www.ncbi.nlm.nih.gov/pmc/articles/PMC5101798/. Accessed 5, January 2021.

Jen Thomas. "GERD: Facts, Statistics, and You." Healthline, https://www.healthline.com/health/gerd/facts-statistics-infographic. Accessed 13, December 2020.

Joel E. Richter and Joel H. Rubenstein. "Presentation and Epidemiology of Gastroesophageal Reflux Disease." US National Library of Medicine National Institutes of Health, https://www.ncbi.nlm.nih.gov/pmc/articles/PMC5797499/. Accessed 13, December 2020.

Laura Dan. "The Standard American Diet: What You Need to Know and How to Break the Status Quo." FullScript.com, https://fullscript.com/blog/standard-american-diet. Accessed 14, February 2021.

M. S. Chorti et. al. "Knowledge of primary care doctors about laryngopharyngeal reflux disease." Royal Belgian Society for Oto-Rhino-Laryngology, Head and Neck Surgery. http://www.b-ent.be/en/knowledge-of-primary-care-doctors-about-laryngopharyngeal-reflux-disease-13426. Accessed 10, January 2021.

Salynn Boyles. "Study: Acid Reflux on the Rise." WebMD, https://www.webmd.com/heartburn-gerd/news/20111222/study-acid-reflux-prevalence-increasing#1. Accessed 5, January 2021.

"Silent Laryngopharyngeal Reflux (LPR): An Overview." The Voice Institute of NY, http://www.voiceinstitute-ofnewyork.com/silent-laryngopharyngeal-reflux-lpr-an-overview/. Accessed 13, December 2020.

Takahisa Yamasaki and Ronnie Fass. "Reflux Hypersensitivity: A New Functional Esophageal Disorder." US National Library of Medicine National Institutes of Health, https://www.ncbi.nlm.nih.gov/pmc/articles/PMC5628981/. Accessed 10, January 2021.

Takahisa Yamasaki et al. "The Changing Epidemiology of Gastroesophageal Reflux Disease: Are Patients Getting Younger?" US National Library of Medicine National Institutes of Health, https://www.ncbi.nlm.nih.gov/pmc/articles/PMC6175565/. Accessed 13, December 2020.

Tawakir Kamani. "The prevalence of laryngopharyngeal reflux in the English population." PEPTEST, https://www.peptest.co.uk/wp-content/uploads/2018/05/2012-Kamani-et-al-The-prevalence-of-laryngopharyngeal-reflux-in-the-English-population.pdf. Accessed 13, December 2020.

"When does a Hiatal Hernia Require Surgery." DrTurn-quest.com, https://www.dturnquest.com/blog/when-does-a-hiatal-hernia-require-surgery. Accessed 5, January 2021.

Diagnostic Tools

"Diagnosing Acid Reflux Disease." Web MD, https://www.webmd.com/heartburn-gerd/guide/diagnosing-acid-reflux-disease. Accessed 8, September 2020.

"Helicobacter Pylori (H. Pylori) Tests." US National Library of Medicine, medlineplus.gov/lab-tests/helicobacter-pylori-h-pylori-tests/. Accessed 8, September 2020.

Medical Treatments

Annette (Gbemudu) Ogbru. "Antacids." Rxlist.com, https://www.rxlist.com/antacids/drug-class.htm. Accessed 13, December 2020.

Benjamin Ka Seng Thong et. al. "Proton Pump Inhibitors and Fracture Risk: A Review of Current Evidence and Mechanisms Involved." US Library of Medicine National Institutes of Health, https://www.ncbi.nlm.nih.gov/pmc/articles/PMC6540255. Accessed 10, January 2021.

C. Fooks. "Antacids." Drugs.com, https://www.drugs.com/drug-class/antacids.html. Accessed 13, December 2020.

Lynne Eldridge . "Top 10 Cancers Causing Death in Men." Verywell Health. https://www.verywellhealth.com/top-can-cers-causing-death-in-men-2248874. Accessed 10, January 2021.

"H2 Blockers." About GERD, https://www.aboutgerd.org/medications/h2-blockers.html. Accessed 13, December 2020.

Gottfried Lemperle. "Gastroesophageal Reflux Disease (GERD): An Overview of Current Minimal-Invasive Treatment Potentials." Biomedical Science & Research, https://biomed-grid.com/fulltext/volume2/gastroesophageal-reflux-disease-gerd.000619.php. Accessed 13, December 2020.

Ilmo Kellokumpu et.al. "Quality of life following laparo-scopic Nissen fundoplication: Assessing short-term and long-term outcomes." US Library of Medicine National Institutes of Health, https://www.ncbi.nlm.nih.gov/pmc/articles/PMC3699043/. Accessed 10, January 2021.

Irvin Modlin. "Historical perspectives on the treatment of gastroesophageal reflux disease." Gastrointestinal Endoscopy Clinics, https://www.giendo.theclinics.com/article/S1052-5157(02)00104-6/fulltext. Accessed 13, December 2020.

Michael Kerr. "H2 Receptor Blockers." Healthline, https://www.healthline.com/health/gerd/h2-blockers. Accessed 13, December 2020.

Patricia Raymond. "Prokinetics and Acid Reflux." Dummies.com, https://www.dummies.com/food-drink/special-diets/acid-reflux-diet/prokinetics-and-acid-reflux/. Accessed 13, December 2020.

Sarah Lewis. "The Top 50 Drugs Prescribed in the United States." Health Grades, https://www.healthgrades.com/right-care/patient-advocate/the-top-50-drugs-prescribed-in-the-united-states. Accessed 13, December 2020.

"William Beaumont." Wikipedia, https://en.wikipedia.org/wiki/William_Beaumont. Accessed 13, December 2020.

Underlying Root Causes

Erika Ebbel. "Your Gut Microbiome: The Most Important Organ You've Never Heard Of | Erika Ebbel Angle | TEDxFargo," Tedx Talks, https://youtu.be/B9RruLkAUm8. Accessed 9, February 2021.

James Helm. "Acid Neutralizing Capacity of Human Saliva." American Gastroenterological Association, https://www.gastrojournal.org/article/S0016-5085(82)80286-2/pdf. Accessed 13, December 2020.

Jayne Leonard. "What is hypochlorhydria?" Medical News Today, https://www.medicalnewstoday.com/articles/322491. Accessed 9, February 2021.

Markus Goldshmiedt. "Effect of Age on Gastric Acid Secretion." American Gastroenterological Association, https://www.gastrojournal.org/article/0016-5085(91)90724-Y/pdf. Accessed 9, February 2021.

Mike Varshavski, "Probiotics Benefits + Myths | Improve Gut Health | Doctor Mike." Doctor Mike, https://youtu.be/scDmziIwUEY. Accessed 9, February 2021.

N.A. Tobey. "What regulates bicarbonate secretion by esophageal submucosal glands?" World Organization for Specialized Studies on Diseases of the Esophagus, http://www.oeso.org/OESO/books/Vol_5_Eso_Junction/Articles/art146.html. Accessed 13, December 2020.

Pruthvi Revaiah et al. "Risk of small intestinal bacterial overgrowth in patients receiving proton pump inhibitors versus proton pump inhibitors plus prokinetics." US National Library of Medicine, https://www.ncbi.nlm.nih.gov/pmc/articles/PMC6206996/. Accessed 13, December 2020.

Siri Carpenter, "That gut feeling." American Psychological Association, https://www.apa.org/monitor/2012/09/gut-feeling. Accessed 9, February 2021.

"The Human Microbiome." Washington.edu, https://depts.washington.edu/ceeh/downloads/FF_Microbiome.pdf. Accessed 1, January 2021.

Phase II: Restore

Annette McDermott. "Can You Use Apple Cider Vinegar to Treat Acid Reflux?" Healthline, https://www.healthline.com/

health/digestive-health/apple-cider-vinegar-for-acid-reflux#other-treatments. Accessed 13, December 2020.

Dr. Eric Berg. "What is Betaine HCL? (And How to Use It)." Dr. Eric Berg DC, https://youtu.be/Jc1y0tfwWlo. Accessed 13, December 2020.

Dr Lenard Wright, "Why Stomach Acid Is Good for You: Natural Relief from Heartburn, Indigestion, Reflux and GERD." Harmony, January 24, 2017

Dr Michael Ruscio, "Betaine HCl: How To Take This Digestive Aid for Low Stomach Acid." DrRuscio.com, https://drruscio.com/betaine-hcl/. Accessed 14, February 2021.

"How to Support Optimal Stomach Acid for Good Digestion" Carolina Total Wellness, http://www.carolinatotalwellness.com/blog/index.php/2019/04/01/how-to-support-optimal-stomach-acid-for-good-digestion/. Accessed 13, December 2020.

Jayne Leonard. "Does apple cider vinegar help with acid reflux?" Medical News Today, https://www.medicalnewstoday.com/articles/324034#other-home-remedies-for-acid-reflux. Accessed 13, December 2020.

Noora Alakulppi. "Apple Cider Vinegar for Bloating and Digestive Issues." Dr. Ruscio, https://drruscio.com/apple-cider-vinegar-bloating-digestive-issues/. Accessed 13, December 2020.

Reagan Young. "HOLIDAY MEALS DON'T HAVE TO BURN. TRY TAKING BETAINE HCL FOR ACID REFLUX." Health Nut Nutrition, https://www.healthnutnutrition.com/blog/betaine-hcl-to-prevent-acid-reflux. Accessed 13, December 2020.

Ninja Tips & Tricks

Jennifer Warner. "Yogurt: An Antidote to Bad Breath?" WebMD, https://www.webmd.com/food-recipes/news/

20050310/yogurt-antidote-to-bad-breath. Accessed 10, January 2021.

Kerri-Ann Jennings. "How Magnesium Can Help You Sleep" Healthline, https://www.healthline.com/nutrition/magnesium-and-sleep. Accessed 14, February 2021.

Epilogue

I sincerely hope you found value in this book. Even more so I hope you find recovery from this illusive disease. Please let me know by leaving an honest review. It motivates me to continue providing content and helping others, like us, who have unwittingly fallen into the reflux cycle.

If you are still working through your recovery, you may want to join my mailing list for other helpful tips. I continue to research and learn as I work with the thousands of individuals who visit my site. No doubt, there are methods in this book that will not work for everyone due to other illnesses, allergies, or complications. In those cases, current and future resources on my site TheAcidRefluxGuy.com may be helpful.

Acknowledgement

Another thanks to my beautiful wife who recommended a complete restructuring of the content in this book. It has no doubt contributed to improving clarity of this text and its many derivatives down the line.

Special thanks to our dear friend Adele for her helpful suggestions, for editing, and finding my many grammatical blunders.

Thanks to Gina, part of my advanced reader team, for the suggestion to expand sections on gut health. This topic will likely be the subject of my next book.

Last, but not least, I want to thank Erin, Saundra, Taylor, Garcia, and Jace for providing and allowing me to use their testimonials for this book.

Praise for Author

"I came across your website and now I follow you on Instagram. Thank you for all your valuable information! I've been struggling for years. Got so bad and such weird symptoms I went to Samsun clinic in Santa Barbara. ENT prescribed PPI's for post nasal drip/LPR. I'm on the third week of your protocol and its life changing. Thanks again." - Erin

"I have LPR...I have been on your program for a few weeks. I am feeling so much better. I finally have a little bit of hope now. I also got my husband started on it and he's feeling much better too. It means so much! I share your insights with friends as well. You are really improving people's lives! I just wanted to say thank you. :)" – Saundra

"I just want to point out that I'm a nurse and I think that the information you are providing and the people you are helping is amazing. Long term PPI use comes with many consequences and having other natural alternatives is key, so thank you!" – Taylor

"Since I started your program my regurgitation has reduced significantly. Little to no heartburn. I feel like my sleep is way better now. I'm having dreams once again. I have been off pantoprazole almost 2 months now thank God. That stuff made me feel horrible." – Garcia

"I was diagnosed with GERD at 16, and controlled it for the first 10 years by avoiding trigger foods - dairy, fat, simple carbohydrates, acidic foods - and frequently just suffering with the acid reflux that came with indulging in comfort foods. Then in my early 20s, I had other digestive issues come up which exacerbated my GERD symptoms and led to mounting damage of my esophagus, giving me migraines and all sorts of upper esophageal reflux symptoms. I was prescribed long-term PPI use. It seemed like a miracle at the time, as I could suddenly enjoy all foods and beverages without acid reflux. Unfortunately my other digestive issues continued and I eventually had to cut out all my old GERD triggers anyway, and then some.

Here I am 18 years later, reading about the dangers of long-term PPI use and researching ways to work more skillfully with my digestive system and hopefully gain freedom from an incredibly restrictive diet. I quit taking omeprazole on December 7th. This is my 3rd or 4th time trying to get off PPIs. About a week off the PPI this time arounds, the GERD symptoms started to come back with a vengeance in spite of keeping to what I thought was a GERD-safe diet.

I finally got an appointment with my doctor who told me that rebound reflux was something she'd never seen or heard of in her clinical practice and advised me to try using H2 blockers as it seemed I was simply a lifelong GERD sufferer and the H2 blockers had lesser consequences than the PPIs.

I took one last look around the web to see if there was anything I had not tried yet, and came across your website. To my incredulity, using your method, I experienced immediate relief of the burning in my throat, the swelling in my palate, face and sinuses, and the other symptoms I had been suffering through.

I am so incredibly grateful to feel like my system is finally finding rebalance! Better than continuing the downward PPI/

H2 blocker spiral of suppressing my body's natural digestive processes. Thank you for putting the guide together and for writing a book that will go more in-depth for all those of us who can benefit from your knowledge and experience!" - Jace

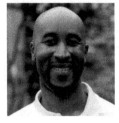 Don suffered reflux for +15 years. Ultimately his symptoms escalated to the point where they could not be managed by medication. Dissatisfied with medical advice, he researched the root causes of acid reflux. By addressing the root causes, he was able to eliminate his reflux for good!

Printed in the USA
CPSIA information can be obtained
at www.ICGtesting.com
CBHW070326180924
14636CB00009B/620